Jim Shimp

AMERICAN RED CROSS

P9-CFR-040

FIRST AID TEXTBOOK

Prepared by The American National
Red Cross for the Instruction of
First Aid Classes

FOURTH EDITION REVISED 1957
WITH 269 ILLUSTRATIONS

41st PRINTING

FEBRUARY, 1973

DOUBLEDAY & COMPANY, INC.
Garden City, New York

THE MISSION OF THE RED CROSS

The American Red Cross is the instrument chosen by the Congress to help carry out the obligations assumed by the United States under certain international treaties known as the Geneva or Red Cross Conventions. Specifically, its Congressional charter imposes on the American Red Cross the duties to act as the medium of voluntary relief and communication between the American people and their armed forces, and to carry on a system of national and international relief to prevent and mitigate suffering caused by disasters.

All the activities of the American Red Cross and its chapters support these duties.

Nationally and locally the American Red Cross is governed by volunteers, most of its duties are performed by volunteers and it is financed by voluntary contributions.

The First Aid program of the American National Red Cross, for which this book is a teaching text, stems from the Congressional charter provision that the organization shall devise and carry on measures for relieving and preventing suffering.

 2

PREFACE TO THE 4th EDITION 1957

Constant medical research brings with it changes that affect first aid advice given to the general public by the American Red Cross. Therefore, the need to revise the first aid textbook at regular intervals is readily apparent. Since accident prevention is an important part of first aid education, there is a need to review preventive measures recommended as well as remedial advice. This book has been prepared so that the reader can easily obtain the desired information, both preventive and remedial, for safer living.

The American Red Cross wishes again to express deep appreciation to the committees on Medicine and Surgery and to appropriate subcommittees of the Division of Medical Sciences, National Academy of Sciences, National Research Council, for reviewing the remedial advice contained in this book.

The basic manuscript was prepared by Carl J. Potthoff, M.D., M.P.H., University of Nebraska College of Medicine. Administrative, medical, and technical staffs of the Red Cross helped prepare this edition as they have previous editions since the inception of the program in 1909.

First aid instruction continues to exert positive influence, as a separate subject or as an integrated part of on-going safety programs in industries, schools and colleges, youth organizations, and city, state, and federal government. It is a "portable" safety program.

The Federal Civil Defense Administration urges the public to take first aid training as a basic step for personal survival.

The Federal Civil Defense Administration is cooperating with the American National Red Cross and other volunteer organizations throughout the country to extend first aid training to every household. First aid training is a valuable home and community resource at all times. Such training helps the individual to prevent accidents and to care for himself and his immediate family when accidents do occur. It is invaluable in any kind of disaster. The training equips you to know what to do and what not to do for the injured until medical help can be obtained.

In the event of nuclear attack on this country, survival may very well depend on what everyone does for himself, one's family or neighbor during the first critical hours following such an attack.

The advent of the thermonuclear age has not changed the responsibility imposed on the American National Red Cross by Congress granted charter. A major portion of ANRC responsibility is to train people in first aid and each Red Cross chapter has the volunteer organization to carry on such a volunteer training program.

I urge every family member to accept this basic civil defense responsibility, to support his vital requirement toward home security and be ready when needed in time of a national emergency.

ADMINISTRATOR
FEDERAL CIVIL DEFENSE ADMINISTRATION

CONTENTS

CONTENTS

STANDARD
FIRST AID
THEORY AND SKILLS

CHAPTER I

THE WHY AND HOW OF FIRST AID

Definition of First Aid

First aid is defined as the immediate and temporary care given the victim of an accident or sudden illness until the services of a physician can be obtained.

First aid commences with the steadying effect upon the stricken person when he realizes that competent hands will help him. The victim suddenly has new problems and needs. Often he cannot think well temporarily. Events may seem unreal and remote. His mind may be dull. The emotional reaction associated with a serious accident subsides only gradually. Therefore first aid is more than a dressing or a splint. It relates to the victim's mind and spirit as well as to his physical injuries. Its contributions include the well-selected word of encouragement, the expression of willingness to help, and the uplifting effect of the first aider's evident capability. The thoughtful suggestions made to solve the immediate problems, the information given concerning nearby physicians and hospitals, the telephone call to summon medical help or an ambulance or to notify a relative—these too are first aid.

The good first aider deals with the whole situation, the person, and the injury. He knows what not to do as well as what to do. Thus he avoids the errors so commonly made through well-meant but misguided efforts. He confines his procedures to what is necessary, recalling that the handling of injured parts should be kept to a minimum.

The Value of First Aid Training

Value to self

Although many people study first aid in order to help others, the training primarily helps the student himself. It enables him to give proper immediate care to his own injuries. If he is too seriously injured to help himself, he may be able to direct others toward proper care. He need not entrust his injured body to the first aid knowledge of random passers-by.

First aid training also helps the student by developing his safety consciousness. Most people recognize the gravity of our accident problem. Their efforts toward safety, however, may be occasional and hit-or-miss rather than a part of a carefully organized plan developed by them for safe living. The first aid course sharpens the desire for safety, shows how accidents occur, and focuses attention upon

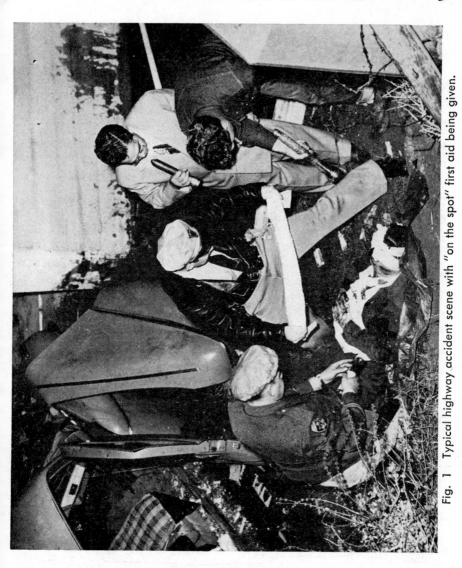

Fig. 1 Typical highway accident scene with "on the spot" first aid being given.

many specific ways to avoid accidents. A good way to guide anyone toward safety is to have him take a first aid course.

Value to others

Having studied first aid, one is more likely to assist family members wisely if they are stricken, to give them some instruction in first aid, and to promote among them a reasonable safety attitude. While the principal benefits are to the student and his family, they extend farther, usually, to co-workers, acquaintances, and strangers. There is always an obligation on a humanitarian basis to assist the stricken, the helpless.

Value in civil defense

First aid training is recognized as an important aspect of civil defense. In case of catastrophe, with medical and hospital service curtailed, citizens must rely largely upon themselves for a time, caring for their own injuries and for those of others. Possession of first aid knowledge is a civic responsibility.

Value in fostering safety consciousness

Disabling accidents, severe enough to cause loss of time from the usual duties for at least one day after the day of injury, occur annually in from one-fifth to one-fourth of our family units. After the first year of life, all through childhood and early adulthood, accidents are the commonest cause of death; thereafter they are *one* of the leading causes. The rate is about twice as high among males as females, with many wage-earners affected. The annual costs for medical and hospital service and direct property damage alone total slightly less than one percent of national personal income. When all wage losses and insurance costs are added, the total is about three percent. Such costs, year after year, greatly affect welfare expenses, and rehabilitation needs. They reflect the fact that many daily serious accidents represent an enormous expense and a large number of personal tragedies.

How can first aid help us avoid accidents? Some reasons have already been given. When we spend some hours studying fractures, head injuries, and burns, we appreciate with more force what it means to suffer injury. Thereafter safety programs seem more important and we personalize their message better. Thus first aid training fosters forcefully the safety consciousness that we all need.

General Directions for First Aid

Most accidents are minor and the first aid needed is obvious to a trained person. In case of serious injury, the following sequence of action is usually applicable: give the urgently necessary first aid, have the victim lie down, check for injuries, plan what to do, and carry out the indicated procedures.

Give urgently necessary first aid

Act quickly for injuries where each second of delay is important: (a) severe bleeding, (b) stoppage of breathing where artificial respiration helps, and (c) poisoning. The proper first aid will be described later. While the first aider's time and attention are devoted to the patient, someone else should go or call for a physician.

Certain other injuries require prompt help—severe burns, for example—but the *immediate* danger to life is not so great. The urgent cases are seldom encountered; they can usually be recognized and the first aid requirements are relatively simple. With most serious accidents, the first aider commences with the next step.

Keep the victim lying down

Protect him from unnecessary manipulation and disturbance. Do not heat the patient but keep the body temperature from falling. Blankets beneath are usually more important than above, but there is hazard in placing them before you know where the injuries are.

Check for injuries

Your clues are the story of what happened, the victim's reactions after the accident, his own ideas about his injuries, and your findings upon examination. The direction and extent of examination should be guided by the kind of accident and the needs of the situation. *Have a reason for what you do.* If the urgent first aid has been given and the patient is properly protected pending early arrival of a physician, a detailed examination is unnecessary. If you must move the victim even a short distance before the physician comes, you should first learn what body parts are injured so that you can support them adequately during the transfer.

Suppose, however, you must carry through with first aid and perhaps transport the victim. Here you must check carefully for injuries. Sometimes the task is simple because it clearly involves a single exposed part, or because, by the nature of the accident, there is no possibility of fractures, lacerations, and the like. An example is poisoning. In other cases you recognize that any body part may be injured and require attention. These cases are the accidents caused by force: for example, traffic accidents, falls, gunshot wounds, blows. With them, you should assure yourself, through consideration of the above-mentioned clues, about every body part—the head, neck, trunk, each extremity in turn. Remember always to consider head injury and back injury. With each part, think of surface injury, of fractures, and of internal organ injury. In addition, note the patient's general condition and state of consciousness.

Surface injuries are readily evident. Fractures and internal organ injuries present greater difficulties. Visual evidence may be lacking with the former and almost always is with the latter. Therefore your objective in checkup for them is simple: find what body parts are, or possibly may be, injured. Your first aid should aim to keep these parts immobile.

Checkup for injuries is far more accurate when the body part is exposed. Such exposure may be possible in the home. Utmost caution should be used when clothing is removed, lest added injury result. In public places, with strangers as victims, exposure of body parts that possibly may be injured is not generally advisable. In such case you must act in the light of such knowledge as you can obtain from the story of the accident, the victim's ideas and reactions, and whatever checkup you can make. When in doubt about a body part, keep it from twisting, bending, and shaking, and do not jackknife the patient. Do not pick him up by head and heels.

Plan what to do

Get a physician or ambulance or obtain medical advice by telephone. This should be one of the first moves. Discuss the problem with responsible relatives or friends of the victim who are at hand or briefly with the victim. If helpers are needed, instruct them carefully in their duties.

Carry out the indicated first aid

Knowing what to do presents few difficulties, once the nature and location of the injuries are learned. Do not attempt to save time and effort by using second-best methods of first aid for this person entrusted temporarily to you in his distress. First, stop profuse bleeding and determine whether artificial respiration is necessary. After that, one may take time for a more general examination.

Selected additional pointers

Find all the injuries. The checkup is often incomplete or sketchy after the first injury is found—especially if it is a major injury.

Give first aid to minor as well as major injuries. For example, a common error upon finding a fracture of a large bone and one of a small bone is to splint only the large bone.

Do not give fluids to an unconscious or partly conscious person, because they may enter the windpipe. Do not attempt to rouse an unconscious person by shaking him, talking, or shouting.

Following injury, do not lift a gasping person by the belt. This is done very often and may aggravate injuries of the back or internal organs. Gasping is not always caused by

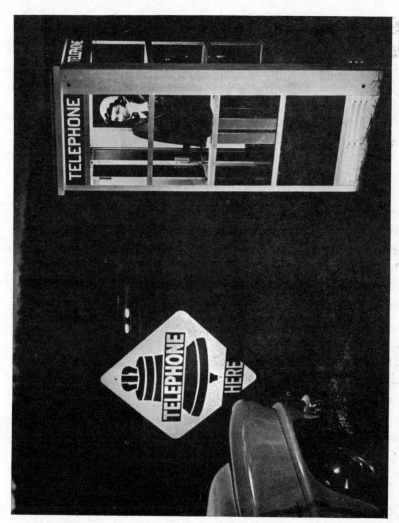

Fig. 2   Telephones are available along main highways to summon medical assistance.

insufficient oxygen but may be due to injury of back or chest.

With indoor accidents, use judgment about opening windows when weather is cold except when noxious gases are present and may have caused the accident. Indoors or out, the victim has enough air, and cold air may be too chilling.

Be reluctant to make statements to the victim and bystanders about the injuries. It is not the first aider's province to diagnose, evaluate, and predict. Upon questioning from the victim, you can answer that you would rather have the physician give information. Helpers must be given necessary information, however.

Obtain the victim's name and address. When calling for a physician or ambulance, be sure to give the exact location of the injured person, and such information as you have concerning the nature of the injuries. Be sure that the physician or ambulance driver knows where to go. Take advantage of the telephone call to obtain good advice concerning first aid. To avoid missing questions or advice, wait until the physician or driver hangs up.

Reassure the victim by telling him what first aid steps you are going to take and how they will help him.

If the victim is unconscious, loosen clothing about his neck. If there is no fracture turn the patient on his side, maintaining this position by flexing the leg or legs, and place a pillow under the head so that secretions may drool from the corner of the mouth. This will usually allow good respiration.

CHAPTER II

WOUNDS

(**Objective** *To protect the wound from contamination and control bleeding.*)

Definition

A wound is a break in the skin or mucous membrane. It is caused by force and usually extends into the underlying tissue. Wounds may be classified into four types.

1. Abrasions, made by rubbing or scraping. Floor burns or scuff burns, although called burns, are true wounds.
2. Incised wounds, sharp cuts that tend to bleed freely.
3. Lacerated wounds, jagged or irregular wounds, often associated with much tissue damage.
4. Puncture wounds. A tack, run through the skin, makes a typical, small puncture wound.

Wounds are subject to infection and bleeding. Deep wounds may be complicated by injury to internal organs and by fractures.

Prevention

Wounds are common accidental injuries, but many can be prevented. Some measures might include:

[11]

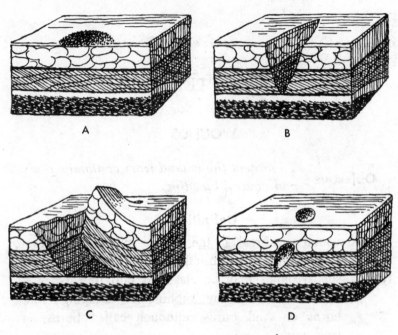

Fig. 3   Four types of wounds
A. Abrasion   B. Incised   C. Lacerated   D. Punctured

1. Keep firearms and ammunition under lock and key.
2. Keep knives, scissors, and other sharp implements in a special storage place, well out of reach of small children.
3. Caution children about running while carrying sharp instruments and about running against glass doors.
4. Put razor blades in a closed container where children cannot find them.
5. Take special care when using knives or other sharp

implements. Always hand a knife to another person with the point turned away from the recipient.

6. Be especially careful in handling such equipment as power mowers or power tools. Follow instructions carefully.

7. Make sure that broken glass is swept up promptly.

Infection

The growth of harmful germs in a wound constitutes a wound infection. The germs destroy tissue about them. Some kinds liberate poisons (toxins) that are carried throughout the body, causing fever, and systemic injury.

Germs are everywhere about us in great numbers. Some kinds are not harmful to man. Few can penetrate the intact skin; but when a break, however tiny, occurs in the skin, there is danger of infection. The body, like virtually all objects about us, has a coating of germs. Therefore a penetrating object carries in its own supply of germs and also pushes some from the skin and perhaps the clothing into the wound.

Evidence of infection does not appear at once after injury, because the germs need some time to grow and multiply. The evidence usually appears from two to seven days or more later. The wound area becomes tender, red, warm, and swollen; sometimes pus appears. Pus consists of white blood cells, germs, and tissue debris. White blood cells, like certain body chemicals, aid in fighting germs. Sometimes red streaks extend from the wound up the arm or leg, and there may be tender nodules (small lumps) in the armpit or groin. These indicate that certain drainage channels, the lymph vessels, are also infected and show that the infection is spreading. Fever and headache are often associated with infected wounds.

The tiniest wound permits entrance of thousands of germs. Any wound, no matter how small, should have adequate attention. The man who boasts that he never has had an infection has merely been fortunate. In the past, he happened to have resistance against the germs that entered his wounds. Tomorrow he may meet a different variety. However, self-treatment is occasionally resorted to.

Wounds of the palms, of the lower extremities below the knees, or the face, and those overlying joints involve greater than usual danger. If infection develops in these areas, results may be grave. Diabetics, and those with hardening of the arteries or other circulatory disease, especially should beware of infection in the lower extremities.

First Aid

Wounds in which bleeding is not severe

Home care for minor scratches. The best source of information concerning home care for minor scratches is the family physician. Lacking such advice, the following procedure may be followed if you elect to assume personal responsibility and the risks of home care:

1. Wash your hands thoroughly with clean water and soap.
2. Cleanse the injury thoroughly, using plain soap and boiled water cooled to room temperature or clean running tap water and soap, applying the soap and water with a sterile dressing. Sterile dressings are described below.

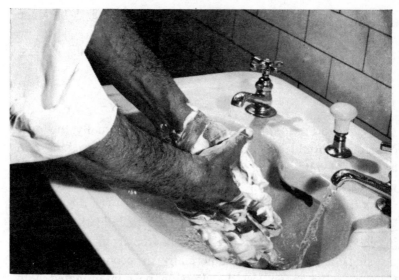

Fig. 4 Wash the hands thoroughly with soap and water.

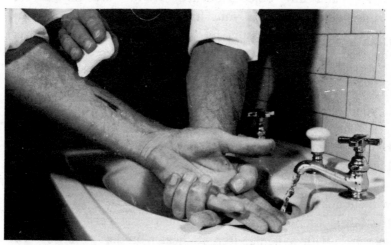

Fig. 5 Washing a small cut.

3. Apply a dry sterile or clean dressing, and bandage it snugly into place.
4. Tell the patient to see his doctor promptly if evidence of infection appears.

First aid preliminary to medical care. Usually the only procedure should be to apply a sterile or clean dressing and bandage it into place. Exceptions are noted with special wounds later. The term "dressing," as used in this textbook, refers to the material that is placed directly over the wound; and "bandage" means the material used to hold the dressing in place. Sterile dressings are entirely free from germs. Such dressings are available commercially in protective packets. Care must be taken lest the dressing be contaminated with germs while you apply it. The hands, the outside of the packet, and any object touched by the dressing harbor germs. Therefore wash your hands first. Upon opening the packet, grasp the dressing by one corner and place it over the wound so that the corner you touched does not overlie the wound. Do not cough or breathe closely upon the dressing. Dressings should be large enough to extend well beyond the wound edges; remember that they may slip.

Then bandage the dressing into place. Bandages should be clean, but not necessarily sterile. They should be snug, but not tight enough to impede circulation.

If sterile dressings are not available, use a clean fabric, with at least four layers over the wound. If possible, treat the fabric to remove at least some of the germs. You can scorch it with a flame, iron it, heat it under close observation in a hot oven, wash it with soap and water and then dry it thoroughly, or expose it for at least ten minutes to the direct rays of the sun. The best method is to boil the fabric for a few minutes, and then dry it. Fluff cotton should not be placed upon a wound; the fibers are hard to remove.

Wounds in which bleeding is severe

The objective is to stop the bleeding at once, always if possible with *pressure* directly over the wound with a cloth.

You may save a life by controlling hemorrhage. If a large blood vessel is cut, blood loss may be sufficient within less than a minute to cause death; but in most cases, body protective mechanisms soon cause some diminution of bleeding. Sometimes, when a limb is severed by a crushing force, there is surprisingly little bleeding, because the cut ends are closed by the force and clots form. The ends may re-open when the blood pressure rises again. The average-size male has about six quarts of blood, the female somewhat less in proportion to size. Adults can withstand readily the loss of a pint, the amount usually taken for transfusion purposes. Loss of over a quart of blood may be serious, especially in the aged and debilitated.

Direct pressure. Most external bleeding can be controlled by applying pressure directly over the wound. Use a clean cloth or a part of the clothing in real emergencies. The cleaner and more nearly sterile the cloth the better in preventing infection. Application of the bare hand may be necessary for quick action in stemming a major blood loss until effective cloth material can be brought to use. After the bleeding has been controlled, apply additional

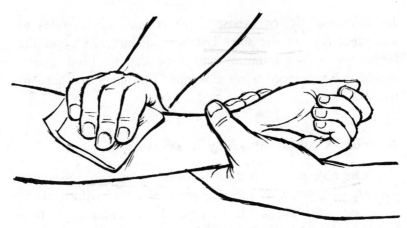

Fig. 6   Direct pressure on the wound.

layers of cloth to form a good-sized covering, and then bandage snugly or firmly. Do not remove the dressing. If blood saturates the dressing, apply more layers of cloth, and perhaps tighten the bandage directly over the wound.

Pressure to the supplying vessel. For especially quick action, in some cases you can use your fingers or the heel of your hand to press the supplying vessel against the underlying bone. Such pressure causes the bleeding to diminish, but does not stop it entirely. Meanwhile you or your assistants can start measures to apply pressure directly over the wound, as described above.

There are only two points on each side of the body where pressure against the supplying vessel is of occasional practical use: (1) Pressure on the inner half of the arm, midway between the elbow and the armpit, compresses the main vessel against the bone there and diminishes bleeding in upper extremity below the point of pressure; (2) pressure applied just below the groin on the front, inner half

3- WAYS to stop Bleeding
1 Direct pressure
2 Pressure Points
3 Turniguet

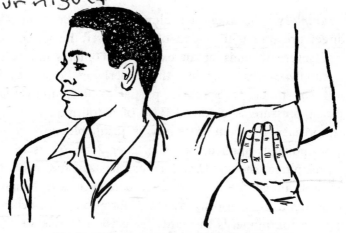

Fig. 7 Finger pressure on brachial artery.

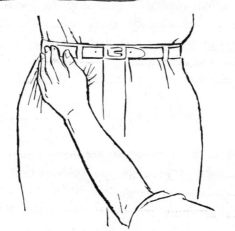

Fig. 8 Hand pressure on femoral artery. →

of the thigh compresses the main vessel against the underlying pelvic bone. If pressure is applied, bleeding should
diminish in the extremity below the point of pressure.

PRESSURE Points
1 Front of EAR - SCALP
2 Clavicle - shoulder
3 neck - mouth
4 mandible - face

Summary. Bleeding can almost always be controlled by direct pressure with a pad of cloth over the wound. In case of severe wounds of an extremity, compression of the main supplying vessel against the underlying bone may be helpful for quick, temporary, partial control until cloth for direct pressure is obtained. Use of a tourniquet in case of hemorrhage from an extremity is justifiable only rarely. If a tourniquet is applied for much over 2 hours, its release may precipitate shock. This fact emphasizes the need for promptness in getting a tourniquet patient to the hospital. He deserves a high priority for transportation. The decision to apply a tourniquet is in reality a decision to risk sacrifice of a limb in order to save life.

The principal objective is to stop the bleeding at once. This almost always can be done with a cloth pad held directly over the wound. The first aid steps are these:

1 Stop the bleeding quickly.

2 Bandage firmly into place the cloths used in controlling hemorrhage.

3 If an extremity is involved, elevate it, using pillows or substitutes.

4 If there is delay in obtaining medical care and if the patient is thirsty, give water as tolerated (approximately ½ glass every half hour)—provided there is no penetrating wound of the abdomen or lower chest. Do not give alcoholic drinks.

Internal bleeding

The signs are similar to those for shock, and the first aid is the same. Shock is discussed in a separate chapter.

Sometimes blood comes from the mouth and nose, though no injury is noted in these organs. The bleeding point probably is in the lungs, stomach, within the skull, or the passages related to them. Provide pillows to raise the head and shoulders if there is breathing difficulty. Try to have the patient control vomiting movements. Give no stimulants even though the bleeding ceases. Medical care is urgently needed. If the patient is in shock or unconscious, turn him on his side, with head and chest lower than hips, to prevent aspiration into the lungs.

Nosebleed

Nosebleeds may occur spontaneously or as a result of injury. There may be an underlying disease, such as high blood pressure, but in many cases there is no disease. Some people, particularly in youth, are often affected following activity, colds, and exposure to high altitude. The bleeding usually is more annoying than serious. Occasionally with underlying disease the bleeding is profuse, prolonged, and dangerous.

The person should remain quiet. A sitting position with head thrown back, or a lying position with head and shoulders raised is best. Walking about, talking, laughing, or blowing the nose may cause increased bleeding or resumption of bleeding.

Usually the bleeding area is near the tip of the nose. Pinching the nostrils together puts pressure upon this area. It may be necessary to pack the bleeding nostril lightly and then pinch. It may be necessary to maintain pressure with a small amount of gauze for several minutes, occasionally considerably longer. Sometimes cold wet towels, applied to the face, stop the bleeding.

Special wounds

The following general principles apply to all wounds: prevent contamination, control hemorrhage, and provide protection. Special wounds are considered at greater length in the Advanced Course. However, selected points deserve mention here.

Infected wounds. Infected wounds should have medical care. Do not pinch the wound and do not open the wound with a "sterile" needle that has been passed through a flame. First aid measures include:

1. Provide rest for the patient. Physical activity favors the spread of infection.

2. Immobilize the affected part. Constant motion of infected fingers, hands, feet, or neck, for example, is harmful.

3. Elevation of an infected extremity, by placing pillows beneath, may be of value. Infections of the lower extremities subside more quickly if the patient has complete bed rest than if he is up and about.

4. Sometimes it is impossible to obtain medical help or advice for many hours. In such cases, wet applications may be administered. Use boiled water to which 2 level teaspoonfuls of salt have been added per quart of water. It is safest to use them at room temperature; they may, however, be warm but never hot. Immerse a towel in the solution and wring it out thoroughly to guard against the frequent mishap of burning the patient. Then apply to the infected wound. A

dry towel may be placed outside the wet one. *Observe carefully lest a burn develop.* Remember that although the towel may not seem too hot when quickly handled, it may cause a burn because of the long contact period. The applications may be continued for half-hour periods with alternate free periods of the same length. Test the temperature of the water by your ability to hold the full container in your hand without dis-comfort from the heat.

Gunshot wounds. Always consider the possibilities of fracture and internal organ injury. If the chest is pene-trated, bandage firmly or snugly over the skin injury to prevent entrance and exit of air. B-B shot, embedded in the skin, are extremely difficult to feel or detect. Advise the doctor so that he may have X-rays taken if their presence is suspected. Police must be notified.

Wounds with danger of tetanus. The danger of teta-nus (lockjaw) should be considered in ALL WOUNDS. Puncture wounds, especially those contaminated with barn-yard soil or manure probably have the highest incidence of tetanus but many cases of tetanus result from wounds so insignificant that the patient does not recall them until specifically questioned. The particular need is for medical attention and possible immunization against tetanus. The danger of tetanus illustrates one of the reasons why even the most insignificant wound should be cleansed without delay.

Animal bites. If a person is bitten by a stray animal, call the police, doctor, and veterinarian immediately. The animal should be restrained or prevented from escaping until their arrival. The bites may cause the usual kinds of infections. In addition, the bite of any warm-blooded animal may cause rabies if the animal harbors the germs of this disease. The disease appears to be invariably fatal in man, once it develops. In this country, the dog, and less often, the cat, skunk, fox, wolf, coyote, and other animals, may be infected. Whenever suspicion of rabies danger exists, the patient should have medical attention at once, and if necessary, the immunization treatments to prevent the disease. The dog should not be killed unless it is essential to protect others from being bitten. The dog should be confined and observed, preferably at the facilities of a veterinarian or dog pound for the presence of rabies.

CHAPTER III

SHOCK

(**Objective** *To prevent or reduce shock by keeping the victim lying down and comfortable.*)

Definition

Shock is a term used with many meanings. Of most importance to first aiders is traumatic shock, which is a depressed condition of many of the body functions due to failure of enough blood to circulate through the body following serious injury.

Decidedly different conditions are electric shock, discussed elsewhere in this textbook; insulin shock, caused by an overdose of insulin; the temporary shock of simple fainting; and the psychiatric condition formerly called shell shock.

Causes and Dangers of Shock

Traumatic shock is associated with injury to body tissue from burns, wounds, or fractures. In most instances it is caused by loss of large quantities of blood either exter-

[25]

nally or into the tissues or body cavities. In general, the greater the damage to flesh and bone and the larger the blood loss, the greater the danger that shock will occur.

Shock may be produced or made worse by any manipulation that increases hemorrhage or causes it to recur. Rough handling of the patient should be particularly avoided. The aged and the debilitated do not withstand shock as well as others.

If a person develops shock and remains in it, death may result even though the injury causing the shock would not be fatal otherwise. Therefore, proper first aid to help prevent or to deal with shock is essential when caring for any seriously injured person.

Signs and Symptoms of Shock

The most important evidence is the victim's weakness, coupled with a skin that is pale and moist and cooler than it should be.

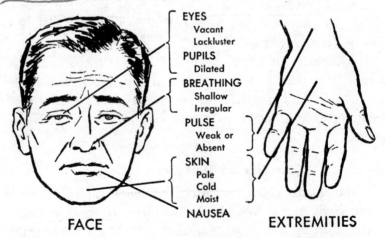

FACE   EXTREMITIES

EYES
Vacant
Lackluster
PUPILS
Dilated
BREATHING
Shallow
Irregular
PULSE
Weak or
Absent
SKIN
Pale
Cold
Moist
NAUSEA

Fig. 9   Signs of shock.

Beads of perspiration may be noted about the lips, forehead, palms, and armpits. The patient may vomit or complain of nausea. His mental reactions may appear normal at first. Later, he may be restless or lose alertness and interest in his surroundings. Thirst is commonly present.

The pulse is fast but may be weak or impossible to feel. The patient may breathe faster than usual and occasionally take deep breaths. These signs may not appear at once. Especially in cases of severe hemorrhage, they may develop only after an hour or more.

Shock should not be confused with simple fainting. Individuals with minor injuries may faint. Even persons who have not been injured may faint at the sight of a serious accident, particularly if blood is visible. One who has fainted will be pale and often covered with perspiration. He may be nauseated. The pulse will usually be slow. If he is allowed to lie flat, recovery will occur promptly.

Since the evidence of shock may not be present, even when the injuries are severe, the first aider may fail to apply proper measures. The victim may seem alert and react optimistically, but suddenly he may collapse. Sometimes only a few signs of shock are noted, and the first aider may think there is little need for concern. He may even permit transportation of the victim in the sitting-up position. The proper course is simple: give first aid for shock to all seriously injured people.

First Aid for Shock

The same first aid measures apply to both prevention and care of shock.

Position

Keep the patient lying down. The lying-down position favors the flow of a greater amount of blood to the head and chest, where it is needed most. It places less demand upon the body than the sitting or standing positions. It is the most favorable position if there is injury to internal organs and the head, or in case of a fracture. There is one exception to the horizontal position: if there is difficulty in breathing, the patient's head and chest should be elevated.

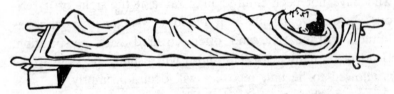

Fig. 10   Position of shock victim when head and chest injuries are absent.

Except as noted below, elevate the lower part of the body if the blood loss is great, or the injury severe. Raise the foot of the bed or stretcher eight to twelve inches. If the victim is on the floor or ground, place pillows or substitutes beneath the lower extremities. This elevation should not be done: (1) if there is a head injury, (2) if breathing difficulty is thereby increased, or (3) if the patient complains of pain when it is attempted, such as pain at a fracture site in the lower extremity or abdominal pain. For lesser injuries, such as a fracture of the wrist, elevation is unnecessary, though not harmful.

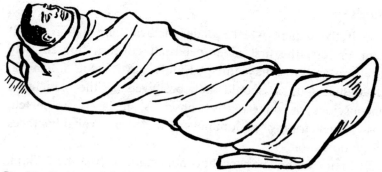

Fig. 11   Position of shock victim when head or chest injuries are present.

Heat

If the victim is lying on the ground or floor, place a blanket beneath him. Cover him only sparingly, according to the temperature of the environment. Do not cause sweating. It is better if he is slightly cool than toasting warm. On warm days little or no surface covering is needed.

Application of external heat by hot water bottles and heating pads is usually harmful in shock. They may be used in cold weather, if sufficient blankets are not available to prevent freezing. If so, use utmost care not to burn the patient. Remember that you test the warm object for only a second or so, whereas it may be in contact with his skin for a long time. Normally his skin will not withstand heat; further, he usually does not recognize that a burn is developing, whether he is unconscious or not. The warm object should have a temperature only slightly above body temperature.

The over-all principle relating to heat in shock is this: do not add heat; simply prevent a large loss of body heat.

Fluids

If the patient will be under medical care within a half hour or less, the first aider need not concern himself with fluids except to allay thirst. Fluids have value in shock. Nevertheless, they should not be given if the patient is unconscious or only partly conscious, if he is nauseated, has a penetrating abdominal wound, or probably faces early operation.

Plain water, neither hot nor cold, is the best fluid. Other drinks may cause nausea, a feeling of fullness, and hiccups. Do not give alcoholic drinks. A set rule concerning the amount of fluid to give cannot be stated, because indi-

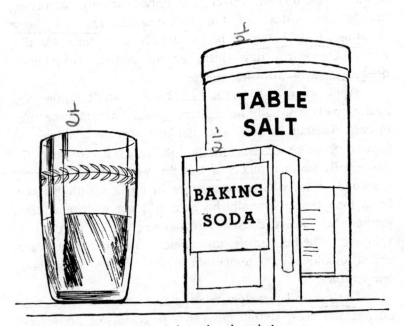

Fig. 12   Salt and soda solution.

vidual cases vary so much. If there will be delay until medical care is available, administer a few sips at first. Observing the patient's tolerance and thirst, increase the amount to a half glass at a time. In case of large blood loss, the patient is usually thirsty and will take drinks at short intervals. Your concern should be to see that he does have fluids, but at such doses and intervals that he does not vomit. If he vomits or is nauseated do not give fluids. If medical care will be unavailable or considerably delayed, give half-glass doses of water, to which has been added one-half level teaspoon table salt and one-half level teaspoon of baking soda per quart, at about 15-minute intervals. Within an hour medical advice should be obtained.

The problem of fluid administration is not great in first aid usually, because the patient will have medical attention fairly soon.

Other measures against shock

The underlying injuries should receive attention; for example, hemorrhage should be controlled and fractures splinted. The victim should not be disturbed by unnecessary questioning, manipulation, and noise. Tactful encouragement should be given. Stimulants such as ammonia or coffee have no value in traumatic shock.

CHAPTER IV

ARTIFICIAL RESPIRATION

Objective ⎧ *To maintain an alternating decrease and* ⎫
⎪ *increase in the expansion of the chest and* ⎪
⎨ *to maintain an open airway through the* ⎬
⎩ *mouth and nose.* ⎭

Definition

Artificial respiration is the procedure for causing air to flow into and from the lungs by mechanical means when natural breathing ceases. Methods that rely upon use of the hands rather than mechanical devices are called manual methods.

Breathing

Need for oxygen

The body does not store oxygen, but needs a continuous fresh supply to carry on the life processes. The products of food oxidation are heat, muscular energy, carbon dioxide (not carbon monoxide), water, and certain other chemicals.

Oxygen must be available to all body cells and is transported to them by the blood. The lungs are the loading zones, and must be ventilated constantly by breathing. Natural breathing is accomplished by increasing and decreasing the capacity of the chest and lungs. Atmospheric air, being under pressure, rushes in and out with the increase and decrease of chest space. As air enters the body, it contains 21 percent of oxygen and 4/100 percent of carbon dioxide. The remainder is largely nitrogen. Air leaving the body has 16 percent oxygen and 4 percent carbon dioxide.

Rate of breathing

The average rate at rest is about sixteen or seventeen times per minute in adults. It is somewhat faster in children, and varies greatly with exercise, excitement, and disease. About a pint of air is inhaled by resting adults with each breath.

The process of breathing

The contraction of chest muscles and the diaphragm causes enlargement of the chest cavity. The diaphragm is a muscular partition forming the floor of the chest cavity and separating it from the abdomen. During the inhalation phase of breathing (inspiration), the muscles of the chest lift the ribs, expanding the chest. At the same time the diaphragm, which is dome-shaped, contracts and descends toward the abdomen. In this way, the chest cavity is increased in size and air flows in. When all the muscles relax, the ribs and diaphragm resume their former position, the chest cavity becomes smaller, and air flows outward. In all manual methods of artificial respiration, the objective is to cause an alternate decrease and increase in the size of the chest cavity. When this is done, air will flow out and in if there is no obstruction.

Conditions Where Artificial Respiration May Be Helpful

Certain accidents and illnesses sometimes cause cessation of breathing even though the body conditions otherwise permit life. In these cases artificial respiration may be life-saving because it supplies oxygen to the body until the normal process can resume.

Artificial respiration does not help if heart action has ceased completely, because in that case the oxygen is not carried from the lungs to the body cells. Artificial respiration must be started promptly after normal respiration ceases. Most persons will die within six minutes or less if breathing stops completely unless they are given artificial respiration; a few might survive somewhat longer. In accident cases, cessation of breathing may go unrecognized for varying periods of time. Precious minutes may have passed. Since the victim may be within seconds of death when the first aider is able to place his hands upon the body, he should immediately seek to obtain an air flow to and from the lungs through any feasible way.

Artificial respiration may be life-saving if administered to non-breathing victims of (1) electric shock, (2) drowning, (3) gas poisoning, (4) poisoning by respiration-depressing drugs, such as morphine, opium, barbiturates, and alcohol, (5) compression of the chest, or for example, by cave-in, (6) choking and strangling, and partial obstruction of the breathing passages. In some cases of gas and drug poisoning, the breathing may be extremely slow and shallow; artificial respiration in such a case may help. It is not essential, though possibly helpful, to time artificial respirations with the patient's efforts. Artificial respiration is of value in poliomyelitis if the breathing mechanism is paralyzed.

Electrocution

In this day of multiple electrical appliances, family members should have basic knowledge about electric flow and home electric dangers. Electrocution may occur from either low voltage (household type) or high voltage currents. The household type offers a more insidious hazard because its danger is often underestimated. A person is more likely to be electrocuted, upon making contact with an electric pathway, if he is simultaneously touching a metal object that directly or by way of a good conduction pathway extends to the ground, if he is standing on a wet floor, or if his skin is damp. The current voltage, the dampness of the skin, and the presence of a good ground determine whether current will pass through the body.

In the home, electric wires are covered with a nonconducting outer covering; when this covering is frayed, one may be exposed directly to the current. Carelessness in allowing numerous cords to be placed under carpets or elsewhere about the room where they may be damaged, or frequent handling of extension cords so that the insulation becomes frayed, often results in potential shorts at switches, outlets, along the wires, or on electrical devices. The point of exposure need be only a tiny fraction of an inch

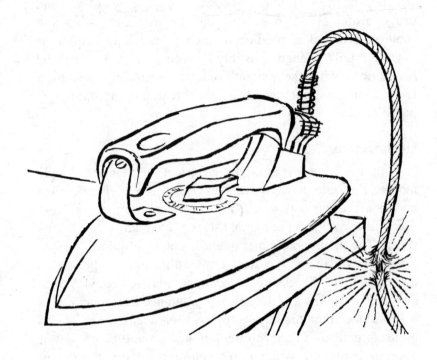

Fig. 13   Replace frayed cords at once.

Prevention. Use only Underwriters' Laboratories (U.L. label) approved electrical equipment. Do not place cords where they may be walked upon. Replace cords that are frayed without delay. Avoid operating electric devices in the bathroom, so far as feasible, and use caution if it is done, keeping in mind the potential dangers of a wet floor, grounded metal pipes, and wet skin. Remember that there may be shorts through virtually any electric device as it becomes older—toasters, electric sewing machines, electric heaters, for example. Keep the hands dry when operating them, and do not touch them simultaneously with grounded metal objects. Do not repair television sets unless you are an expert. Use every precaution with home workshop tools.

Rescue. In case of electric shock, cut off the house switch if possible. Separate the person from the contact by means of a long stick—not one containing sap—or a dry rope or goodly length of dry cloth, being sure that your hands are dry and that you are standing on a dry surface. Out of doors, with high tension wires, your danger in rescue is much greater. Telephone the power company to turn off the currents before you attempt rescue unless you are willing to accept grave risk to your life.

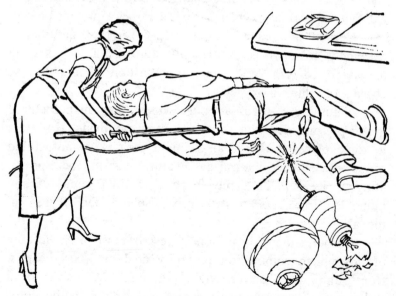

Fig. 14 Roll victim from wire or shut off current.

First aid. Once the rescue is made, give artificial respiration if the victim is not breathing. The body may seem stiff as an effect of the current. It may be necessary to continue the procedure for several hours. If transportation is necessary, consider the possibility of internal organ injuries and fractures.

Poisoning by gas

Asphyxia may occur from breathing air that does not contain sufficient oxygen, or from air containing carbon monoxide or any other toxic gas.

Natural slow oxidation processes sometimes remove the oxygen from the air in wells, cisterns, sewers, mines, and silos. If this air is not changed through ventilation, it will not support life, whether toxic gases are present or not.

Carbon monoxide is an odorless, colorless gas that is extremely toxic. It is present in auto exhaust gases, in manufactured gas, and when combustion occurs in the absence of sufficient oxygen.

Natural gas, used far more widely than manufactured gas at present, does not contain carbon monoxide. However, in some places during peak demand periods, manufactured gas is added to the natural gas. Natural gas may be asphyxiating if it is incompletely burned so that some carbon monoxide forms, or if it largely displaces the oxygen in the air.

Carbon monoxide poisoning results most often because of incomplete combustion in faulty coal or wood heaters, from running gas-driven engines in confined spaces, from the escape of manufactured gas in leaky pipes in the home or in manholes, from open gas jets, and from incomplete combustion of natural or manufactured gas in faulty gas-burning appliances.

In addition to the dangers of asphyxia from carbon monoxide, or from displacement of oxygen by natural oxidation processes or by other gases, there is often an explosion hazard. Combustible gases that accumulate in confined spaces, such as mines, cisterns, basements, and sewers, or in rooms where natural or manufactured gas is free in the air, are explosive in certain concentrations. The explosion may result if a flame is introduced, if static electricity is discharged, or if an electric switch, doorbell, telephone, or other electric device is used.

Prevention. Do not venture into unused places where gases may accumulate. Protect children by filling up or securely covering abandoned wells and cisterns. Never run an automobile or other gas-driven engine in a confined or unventilated space for even a few minutes. Take appropriate precautions with gas used in the home, just as you should with electricity, through safe construction, purchase of good quality apparatus, and immediate repair or removal of defective apparatus. In case of a leak in a gas supply, have the gas company service man search for the leak, meanwhile closing off the gas supply to the building and seeking safety against possible explosion. Keep coal and wood heaters in good condition. Do not use open burners in small, unventilated rooms.

Rescue. In a home, the safest course is to shut off the electric line and the gas line and, if possible, then ventilate the space thoroughly before rescue. Any rescue without such precautions carries great risk. The danger of explosion is usually less if the trouble results from incomplete combustion rather than from leaks or open jets. The danger of asphyxia during rescue varies according to the time of exposure in the affected area. A handkerchief or similar object placed over the face does not screen out noxious gases.

In a garage, danger of explosion is not as great if the victim's mishap was caused by auto exhaust gases. Here you might rescue successfully if you can carry out the victim while holding your breath or taking only a few breaths. If you elect to risk the dangers of explosion and asphyxia by attempting to rescue from a cistern or other dangerous area, tie a rope around your body so that assistants can pull you out if you collapse. Too often risks are taken to rescue a person who is already dead. The best local experts in rescue matters in these cases usually are gas company specialists and firemen. Many police departments have crash trucks and trained crews.

First aid. First remove victim from area and have someone notify the police department as soon as possible to obtain help and special equipment. Give artificial respiration at once if the victim is not breathing or is breathing inadequately. The chance for recovery is much better if some breathing efforts are still being made by the victim. If the respirations are inadequate—irregular, perhaps weak or slow—give artificial respiration at the usual rate. Your efforts will prevail over his feeble efforts. Occasionally you can time an expiration phase with his attempt. Secure oxygen inhalations for him as soon as possible. Recovery may be delayed. Keep the victim recumbent until he is under medical care, meanwhile observing him constantly.

Drowning

Drowning is a leading cause of accidental death. Drownings occur not only among recreational swimmers but also among those who use small watercraft, among youngsters who play along docks and banks of lakes and other bodies of water, among young children who are left in bathtubs or who wander into ponds or canals, and among skaters who break through the ice.

Prevention. It is most important to learn respect for the water—it can be a good friend but a deadly enemy. Everyone should learn to swim. Red Cross chapters and other groups offer swimming instructions in communities throughout the nation. In addition, everyone should know these basic rules of water safety:

1. Never swim alone; make sure someone is nearby who can help in an emergency.
2. Swim at a safe bathing place, preferably supervised by lifeguards.
3. Beware of unfamiliar areas since they may have treacherous currents, deep holes, debris, or other hazards.
4. Don't swim when overheated, overtired, or right after eating.
5. Before diving, make sure the water is deep enough and has no hidden objects.
6. Know your own ability and don't overestimate it; it's hard to accurately judge distance over water.

7. If you are going on a distance swim in open water, have someone accompany you in a boat.

8. Be courteous; consider the safety of others.

If you are using small watercraft, learn to swim well enough to keep yourself afloat. If you don't know how to swim, wear a lifejacket at all times while afloat. Learn to handle your craft. Many Red Cross chapters and other groups offer courses in boating, canoeing, and sailing. If you are using an outboard motor, match the motor to the boat. Don't overload your craft. At least two-thirds of the craft's depth should be freeboard (above the level of the water). If bad weather is threatening, don't go out, and if the weather gets rough while you are out—even if the fish are biting—return to shore. Keep your weight low in the craft at all times. If your canoe or boat upsets or fills with water, it usually will float. Hold onto it for support. Even with a motor attached, it will support the normal number of occupants.

To help prevent drownings around the home, never leave a baby or small child alone in the bathtub, even for a few seconds. If you have a fishpond, put a fence around it to protect small children. Caution children about playing near canals, ponds, quarries, and the like.

In skating, beware of thin ice. A common guide is one inch, keep off; two inches, one may; three inches, small groups; four inches, okay. However, during a midwinter thaw or near the end of the season, even as much as two feet of apparently firm ice may become honeycombed so that slight pressure will break it.

Rescue. Since many drownings occur near shore, you often can help prevent them even if you can't swim. If a

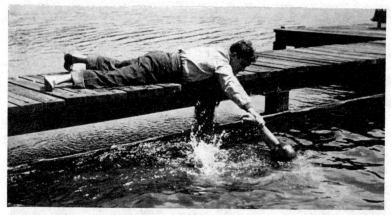

Fig. 15 The hand reach.

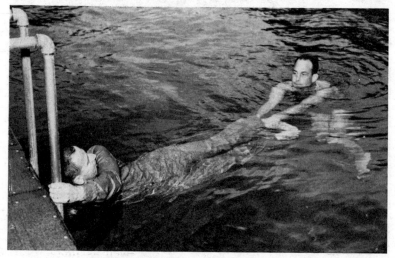

Fig. 16 The leg extension.

bather is in trouble near the dock or side of a pool, lie down
and extend a hand or foot to him; or extend a towel,

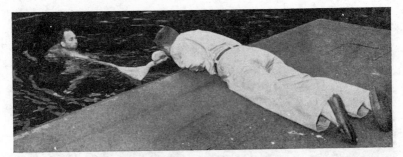

Fig. 17 Extension using towel.

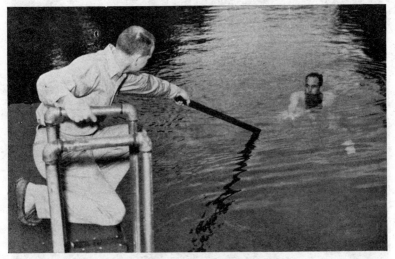

Fig. 18 Extension using pole.

shirt, branch, or pole and pull him to safety; or throw a ring buoy or line. If he is too far from shore for these measures, wade into chest-deep water and extend something to him, or shove a board, plank, or similar object to help keep him afloat while you get more help. If a boat is available, row to the victim and let him grasp the stern, or extend an oar and draw him around to the stern where he can hang on while you row to shore. A swimming rescue should not be attempted except by someone trained in life-saving. Further information can be found in the Red Cross textbook, *Life Saving and Water Safety*.

First aid. If the victim is not breathing, artificial respiration should be started at once, in the boat, or when swimming ashore, using any feasible way to secure compression and relaxation of the chest wall. Then the back pressure-arm lift method can be used as soon as possible, and other first aid measures can be carried out as already described. It is a dangerous waste of time to attempt removing water from the lungs before commencing artificial respiration; little, if any, can be drained out.

Additional Related Information

In cases of recovery, normal breathing usually starts within fifteen minutes after artificial respiration starts, but not infrequently it is delayed, even for hours, because of associated harm from electric shock or depressant drugs or gases. Breathing efforts can be readily detected. Continue your efforts, spaced between those of the victim, until the normal effort is evident.

Sometimes devices called resuscitators are available. These can be adjusted to give artificial respiration, using air or oxygen, to suck out mucous secretions, or to deliver a flow of oxygen while the first aider gives artificial respiration. These should be used only by trained persons. The delivery of oxygen helps especially in case of gas poisoning and when the air passages are partly occluded. It appears that the manual method alone provides the victim with as great a survival chance as does use of the resuscitator except when oxygen is especially needed or when there is excess mucus.

CHAPTER V

POISONING BY MOUTH

Objective *To dilute the poison as fast as possible. Then, except as advised, to induce vomiting.*

Hurry is the word to associate with poisoning by mouth. In most emergencies of this kind, the objective is to dilute the poison by administering fluids, and in most cases to make the patient vomit. There is always a possibility that fluids or gases may be sucked into the lungs when a person is vomiting. If this happens immediate medical care is vital.

Caustic poisons such as lye and strong acids injure the lining of the food passages; the injurious action diminishes when fluids dilute the poison. Obviously, the first aid should be almost instantaneous. Every second of delay causes added injury. Other poisons do not injure the lining, but there is danger that the substance will be absorbed into the system from the digestive tract and cause harm. If the poison can be removed from the stomach by vomiting, the harm will be averted. Once the substance passes well into the intestine, it will usually not be vomited. Therefore, effective first aid must be quick first aid.

[47]

Causes and Prevention

Causes

Poisoning in adults may often be an attempt at suicide. Occasionally an adult is poisoned accidentally by eating contaminated food or by carelessly taking a poison from the medicine cabinet.

Poisoning ranks third as a cause of accidental death in small children. Most young children do not distinguish between what should and should not be eaten. Sometimes they even take extremely ill-tasting or caustic substances.

Poisons commonly taken are:

1. Substances from the medicine cabinet, including drugs, substances intended for external use, pain and headache relievers, sleep-producers, laxatives, antiseptics, and some home permanent wave materials. Almost all prescribed drugs are dangerous if taken in larger-than-directed doses. Aspirin often is taken in poisonous dosage by children.

2. Certain common household supplies, including lye, ammonia, and many other cleansing agents; kerosene and other petroleum products; poisons for use against insects, rodents, and weeds; painting supplies such as turpentine.

Prevention

1. Keep all medicines, household cleansers, disinfectants, exterminators, and other materials well out of the reach of young children.

2. Keep all bottles labeled and always carefully read labels when taking or giving medicines.

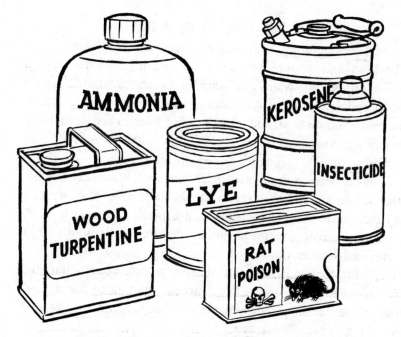

Fig. 19 Common household poisons.

3. Keep poisonous drugs away from other medicine, preferably locked in a separate storage place. Label poisons with large lettering. When their purposes have been served, discard them.

4. Dispose promptly of incompletely used prescription drugs.

5. Educate older children regarding the danger of poisonous substances.

6. Select toys with lead-free paint and keep children from gnawing on surfaces painted with paint containing lead.

Signs and Symptoms

The symptoms of poisoning vary greatly according to the kind and amount of poison taken and the time elapsed since ingestion. Many poisons cause no symptoms until absorbed into the system. Others cause burns in the mouth or cause immediate abdominal pain. There may be nausea, vomiting, visual disturbances, or difficulty in seeing, convulsions or fits, headache, or deep sleep.

The more helpful evidences are (1) information from the victim or an observer, (2) the telltale container, (3) sudden onset of pain or illness in a person previously well, and (4) sometimes burns about the lips and mouth or a revealing breath odor.

The typical story with child poisoning is that the child, usually 1-4 years of age, when unattended for a brief period, tests his environment by tasting and swallowing anything within his reach.

With lye poisoning the poison burns the esophagus (gullet), causing scar formation later. The food passageway becomes constricted and sometimes must be enlarged by means of special instruments or surgery. In kerosene poisoning the child usually gags and vomits. Breath odor is characteristic. Pneumonia is apt to develop later.

First Aid

The label or container should be saved for identification of the poison. The remainder of the ingested substance should also be saved to assist in identifying and estimating the dose.

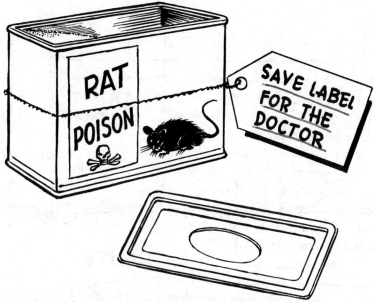

✗ Fig. 20 Save labels for identification.

Give first aid without delay. Obtain medical advice by telephone as quickly as possible concerning antidotes and measures to take. Someone else can telephone while you give first aid. In view of the guilt that parents inevitably feel about the occurrence of poisoning in their children, the first aider should avoid any implication of criticism in his questions concerning the details.

For most cases, proceed as follows:

Dilute the poison. Quickly administer fluid in large amounts—four glasses or more with adults. Water usually is most readily available. Milk protects the digestive tract lining somewhat and slows the absorption of poison. Either or both may be given.

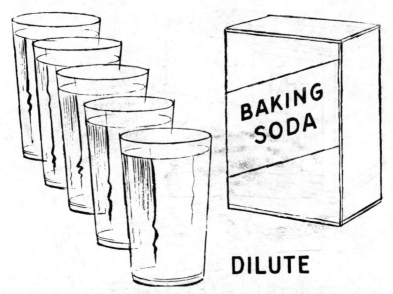

DILUTE

Fig. 21   Four or more glasses of water or milk for adults. Water with several teaspoonfuls of baking soda.

In many cases an important measure is the prompt production of vomiting. When fluids can be administered, the larger the amount of fluid given, the greater the tendency to vomit. Baking soda solution, several teaspoonfuls per half glass of water, is nauseating and may be given persistently with the fluid to induce vomiting. Milk of magnesia is sometimes preferable to baking soda because it produces less gas. Repeat the dilution and induction of vomiting if it appears that poison still remains in the stomach.

If fluid cannot be administered, induce vomiting by (1) holding the child with his hips upon the first aider's lap and his head slightly lower to prevent aspiration of

For alkalis=OH₃

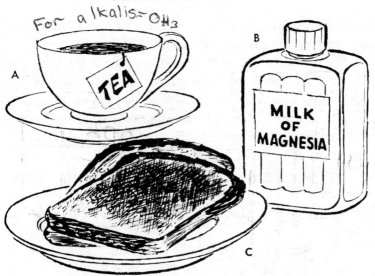

UNIVERSAL ANTIDOTE

Fig. 22   A. 1 part strong tea.   B. 1 part milk of magnesia.   C. 2 parts crumbled burnt toast.

vomitus; (2) using a finger or spoon in the mouth to induce gagging and vomiting.

If the antidote is given on the label, administer it as directed. This can be done with the diluting fluid or after vomiting has occurred. If no specific antidote is known, administer a universal antidote of two parts crumbled burnt toast, one part strong tea, and one part milk of magnesia.

Exceptions to the above procedure

The following exceptions should be noted: (1) poisoning with strong acids, such as carbolic acid, or alkalis, such as lye, (2) strychnine, (3) kerosene, and (4) cases where the victim already is in a coma or clearly has symptoms such as convulsions or exhaustion.

For *strong acids,* dilute quickly with a glass of water and then give milk of magnesia or if not available give baking soda solution, as above described, to neutralize the acid. Do not give enough to cause vomiting. Several glasses may be given. Then give milk, olive oil, or egg white to protect the digestive tract lining.

For *alkalis,* give a glass of water quickly, then vinegar or lemon juice in the diluting fluid to neutralize the alkali. Follow with milk, olive oil, or egg white. Do not cause vomiting.

The only reason for giving plain water first is because it is quickly available.

In strychnine poisoning, the slightest disturbance of the patient may induce convulsions if the poison has entered the system. Give fluids and induce vomiting if only a few minutes have elapsed since the poison was taken; but do not persist long. Get medical care quickly.

In kerosene poisoning, vomiting should not be induced.

If the victim is in a coma, in deep sleep, or clearly has systemic symptoms, it is clear that he took the poison some time before and that all or part of it is already absorbed. In all these cases, keep him warm, do not attempt to give fluids, but seek medical care.

CHAPTER VI

INJURIES TO BONES, JOINTS, AND MUSCLES

(**Objective** *To keep the broken bone ends and the*)
adjacent joints quiet.

Fractures

Definitions

A fracture is a break in a bone. There are two principal kinds, simple and compound. A simple fracture is a
closed fracture not associated with an open wound extending from the skin to the fracture area. When such wound
is associated, the fracture is an open or compound fracture.
When the bone is broken in small pieces, the fracture is
described as a comminuted fracture. A comminuted fracture may be either closed or open.

In an open fracture the wound usually is inflicted by
a broken bone end that tears through the skin and, in most
cases, slips back again. Sometimes it is caused by a missile,
such as a bullet, that penetrates the skin and breaks a bone.
Open fractures are much more serious than closed ones
because the fracture area is always contaminated and infection is virtually certain unless prevented by effective
treatment.

[55]

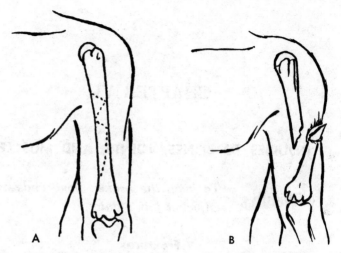

Fig. 23   A. Simple or closed fracture.   B. Compound or open fracture.

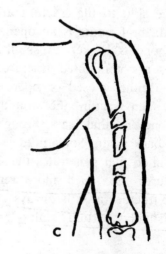

C. Comminuted fracture.

Causes and prevention

Falls and traffic accidents are the commonest causes of fractures. Machinery and missiles also cause many.

Traffic accidents are a leading cause of accidental death and injury. Safety on the highway depends upon many factors—but primarily upon the attitudes of drivers and walkers.

If you are driving be sportsmanlike and courteous. Obey traffic regulations. Keep speed reasonable. Start earlier and drive slower. Don't drive when you drink. Remember, danger increases with darkness; at sundown reduce speed so you're within stopping range of your headlights. Stay in line—don't weave. Don't pass unless there's plenty of room, and never pass on hills or curves. Allow sufficient stopping distance between you and the car ahead. Be extra alert at intersections. Always signal your intention to turn or stop. If weather is bad, don't drive unless you must; if you must, double your care. Keep your car in good condition by having regular checks made of your brakes, lights, windshield wipers, tires, and steering.

If you are walking, cross streets only at crosswalks. Look both ways before crossing. Cross only on proper signal, watching for turning cars. Never go into the roadway between parked cars. If there is no sidewalk and you must walk in the roadway, walk on the left, facing traffic. When walking at night wear or carry something white to help a driver see you.

About three fourths of the deaths from falls in the home occur in those over age 65. Younger people, however, account for some deaths and many nonfatal injuries.

Safe construction, good housekeeping, appropriate education and care in day-by-day living are the facets of a sound preventive program here, as with other accidents. Tension, haste, and fatigue help pave the road to the hospital.

Among steps the homemaker can take to contribute to her family's safety are: Inspect steps, handrails, floors, and carpets to make sure they are in good condition. Make necessary repairs at once. Keep steps and hallways clear. Encourage children to pick up their toys when they have finished playing and provide a good storage place for these items. Use a sturdy ladder or step stool, not a chair, to reach high places. Don't attempt to overreach. Stand on something high enough to enable you to reach easily, and place the ladder so you don't have to overreach to either side. Provide adequate light, especially on stairs. Warn older persons not to walk around in the dark. Make sure a lamp is placed near their bed. To help prevent falls caused by slipping, wipe up spilled grease or water immediately. Make sure small rugs are well anchored.

Signs and symptoms

Since a fracture is an injury beneath the skin surface, it cannot be seen except in occasional cases. The question to answer, therefore, is "Shall I suspect a fracture?" If the answer is "Yes," the proper first aid is to handle as though a fracture were proved.

Evidence is based upon the story of what happened to the victim, the victim's evaluation of his injuries, his reactions after the accident, and the examination. Obtain the story accurately and in detail. Exactly what happened to the person? Was the force sufficient to break a bone?

Regard the evidence so obtained as being only a bit of help. A strong force may not cause a break. On the other hand, surprisingly little force may cause fracture if the leverage is right, or if the victim is elderly or in a weakened condition.

Consider the victim's evaluation. He may have felt the bone break or believes that a break is present. Consider also what he did after the accident and how it affected him. If the victim believes that a fracture is present, always weigh this evaluation strongly. He is frequently correct; but if not, no harm is done by splinting. However, do not rely on the victim's evaluation alone. You must conclude from the overall evidence.

The direct evidences are swelling, tenderness to touch, deformity, and pain on motion. Swelling requires some time to develop. Often the general area overlying the fracture is only slightly tender, but perhaps one small spot will give considerable pain when pressed upon. The fracture probably is directly below. The body part may be out of normal shape. You can detect deformity and swelling in doubtful cases by comparing the part with the other side of the body or with your own body. If the victim tries to move the body or body part so that there is motion, pressure, or tension at the fracture site, he generally has pain. When completely at rest, a fracture usually gives no pain, but a feeling of fullness or swelling. Note, however, that a person *can* move a fractured bone; often he can move the parts below the break with little or no real distress. For example, if the wrist has a fracture, the fingers ordinarily can be flexed, often with no noticeable pain.

In summary, obtain the story of what happened, learn

the victim's evaluation and his reactions, and then check the body carefully for physical evidence. If there is enough overall evidence to base suspicion that a break is present, play the safe side. Be particularly cautious with deep-lying bones: possible breaks of the upper part of the thigh, the upper part of the arm and the shoulder, the backbone, and the pelvis. With them, swelling, tenderness, and deformity may be absent; as clues, you may have only the story of the accident, the victim's evaluation, and his reluctance to move the part. Never test for fracture by having the victim move the part or by attempting to walk upon a possibly broken limb.

If the fracture is compound, there is a wound adjacent to the fracture site. It may be tiny or large. The bone may protrude, but usually it has slipped back if it caused the wound. As with simple fractures, there may be discoloration of the nearby skin because of rupture of blood vessels.

Essentials of first aid

Keep the broken ends quiet.

Keep the adjacent joints quiet. If they bend, the muscles act against the fractured bone, causing motion.

Give first aid for shock.

If the fracture is compound, apply a sterile dressing to the wound. Control hemorrhage by direct pressure. If splints are to be applied in cases where bleeding has been severe, leave a tourniquet loosely in place above the wound so that if bleeding resumes it can be quickly controlled. Do not push a protruding bone back. If splinting and transportation are necessary, the end will slip back when the limb is straightened for splinting.

Fractures, dislocations, and sprains should be treated with an ice bag over the painful area. This limits and reduces swelling and pain.

Preventing motion of fragments. Many methods can be used to prevent movement of the fractured bone. Choice depends, in part, upon the specific bone. Fractures of the extremity bones are usually splinted, but partial immobilization of them is attained if they are placed upon pillows. Transportation of back and pelvis fracture cases by stretcher, door, or cot suffices alone. With fractures in the

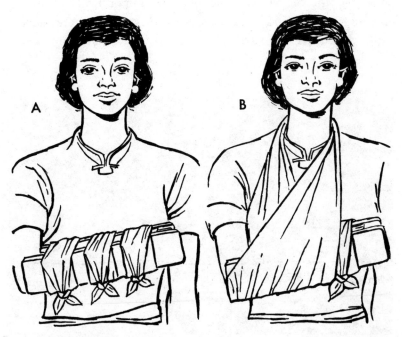

Fig. 24   A. Immobilization of fractured forearm.   B. Arm sling added for further support.

upper extremity, splints may be used; in some cases an arm sling helps immobilize. Breaks of the ribs, face and skull bone need no immobilization device; they are usually "splinted" by adjacent bone and tissue.

Improvised splints should be carefully fashioned or selected. Heavy, irregular, unwieldy items probably do more harm than good. It is wise to keep splints in the home, the automobile, and the workshop.

Specific immobilization methods. Good ways to immobilize specific injuries are described in Section Two. They can serve in case of fracture, internal injury, or severe wounds, all of which benefit from immobilization during the first aid period. Occasionally, other devices and methods, suggested by particular circumstances and the avail-

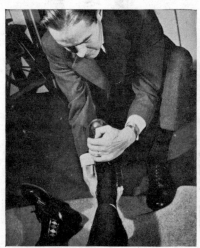

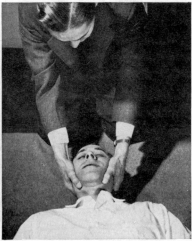

Fig. 25 Holding traction on the lower extremity.

Fig. 26 Holding traction at the head.

ability of materials, may serve as effectively if they keep the injured area of the broken bones and adjacent joints quiet.

Sometimes a limb must be straightened a bit before a splint can be applied. If so, have someone grasp the end of the limb and exert a strong, steady pull, while you place one hand just above the injury and one just below it, thus supporting the site during the straightening process. If the body must be rolled over, it may be best to apply the splint first. If not, support the injury as above described while the patient is being turned. In case of possible back injury, use extreme caution if turning is necessary, being sure to turn the entire body as a unit so that no part twists or turns faster than the other parts. As far as possible, the patient should be kept lying face down.

Additional information about specific injuries and their immobilization is described in the section on practical work.

Head Injury

Knowledge of what to do for this injury is a must for first aiders. The injury is by far the commonest cause of death in traffic accidents and probably also with falls. The essentials are: (1) suspect the injury in any accident due to force and (2) keep the person quiet. Hurried transportation that disturbs and jostles the victim is a grave danger, no matter how desperate his condition seems to be.

Fracture of the skull may or may not be present. The brain injury is the important one; you need not determine whether fracture is present nor give additional first aid for head injury even though fracture is present.

Signs and symptoms

The history of the accident and the presence of swelling or a wound of the head are important clues. Occasionally the pupils of the eyes are unequal in size; a difference, if present, is relatively easy to discern. Bleeding from the nose, an ear canal, or the mouth *sometimes* reflects head injury with a fracture. The bleeding may be only a few drops. Occasionally there is paralysis of one or more extremities. The face may be pale, flushed, or of normal color. The pulse may be slow and full, fast and weak, or normal. Headache is usual and sometimes associated with dizziness.

Unconsciousness or the history that it occurred after the injury, brief or prolonged, point strongly to head injury. Usually the unconsciousness immediately follows the blow. Sometimes, with slow bleeding in the skull, unconsciousness may not begin for a half hour or longer. In the interval the victim may seem normal or dazed, and may walk about.

Whenever the history suggests that the head sustained a forceful blow, whenever there is a history of unconsciousness following possible head injury, and whenever there is headache or dizziness following a blow to the head, give first aid most carefully for head injury.

First aid

If the patient is unconscious, place a small pillow or a substitute under the head. Turn the head toward the side so that secretions may drool from the corner of the mouth.

Loosen clothing about the neck. If the patient is awake he may lie flat.

Whether he is conscious or not, give no stimulants.

If a dressing is needed for a scalp wound, merely lay a large dressing over the injury and then apply a full head bandage.

Sprains

Sprains, which are injuries to the soft tissues surrounding joints, usually result from motion forced beyond the normal range at a joint. The ligaments, muscle tendons, and blood vessels are stretched and occasionally torn or partially torn. The ankles, fingers, wrists, and knees are most often affected. Ankle sprains commonly result when weight is thrown forcefully upon a turned ankle.

Signs and symptoms

Swelling, tenderness, and pain on motion are the signs. Sometimes there is discoloration of the skin over a large area because of rupture of small blood vessels. One cannot distinguish sprains from fractures by the degree of swelling and pain. It should be noted that small chip fractures often occur with the soft tissue injury. The story of what happened, including information concerning the force applied against the joint, is of some help in determining whether the injury is a sprain or a fracture.

First aid

If there is any possibility of fracture, immobilize the part as you would for a fracture. Otherwise, elevate the joint upon pillows or substitutes. Cold, wet applications or an ice bag during the first half hour after injury may retard the swelling. Keep the joint quiet. Do not walk on a sprained ankle until it has a protective support. Always have sprains X-rayed. In case of swelling at a finger joint, as so often happens in athletics, have a physician obtain an X-ray; these injuries frequently are associated with small chip fractures.

Dislocations

A dislocation is a displacement of a bone end from the joint. The surrounding ligaments and other soft tissue always suffer some injury. The fingers, thumb, and shoulder are most often affected. Dislocations are caused by falls and blows usually. Muscular effort may dislocate the arm from the socket in the shoulder blade. Unless properly relocated and cared for, such dislocations may occur repeatedly and cause significant disability.

First aid

Since the signs are similar to those for fractures, the first aider ordinarily should handle the case as a fracture. The part should be kept quiet and medical attention obtained. In the case of fingers and thumb, a splint is not needed if the hand is kept quiet. In the case of the shoulder, apply an arm sling to immobilize the part during transportation. It is unwise to attempt repositioning a shoulder dislocation; the result may be a long-lasting disability. Sometimes, with medical facilities distant, one can pull cautiously upon a dislocated finger in the attempt to bring

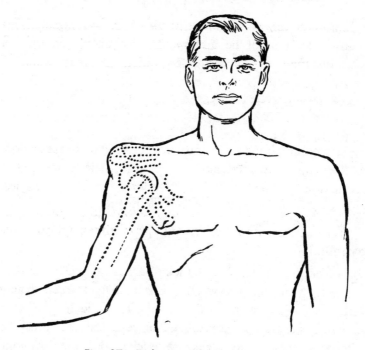

Fig. 27   Dislocation of the shoulder.

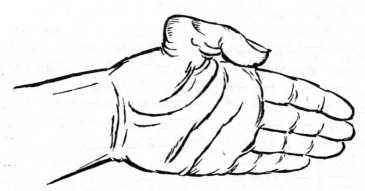

Fig. 28   Dislocation of the thumb.

the bone into place. Do not persist if unsuccessful. This maneuver should not be attempted on a dislocated thumb. The difficulties are much greater and injury may result.

Strains

Strains are injuries to muscles because of overexertion. The fibers are stretched and sometimes partially torn. The more serious strains are those involving the back muscles. These strains are usually caused by lifting.

Prevention

Never try a sudden, quick lift of a heavy object. Never lift from an awkward position. Don't keep trying to lift an object if preliminary efforts indicate the task may cause strain. Use caution when repeated lifts must be made. Use hoists and trucks whenever possible. Anyone can sustain a strain and the effects may persist for a long time.

When it is necessary to lift a heavy object place the feet conveniently close to the object, keep the back straight, get a sure grip with the hands, and attempt the lift gradually, with the legs and thigh muscles bearing the load. In lifting, the amount of force exerted on the structures of the back is approximately eight to ten times greater with the back bent than with the back straight. Both strain and hernia (rupture) are more apt to be avoided if proper methods of lifting are used. Avoid trying to raise a heavy object high; the danger of strain and rupture is too great.

First aid

The first aid consists of rest and warm applications, using wet towels. With a back strain the patient should lie on a hard surface such as the floor rather than on a soft bed.

Some people will disagree as to the first Aid. Some trains want to use ice all the time, as the end result using ice over a long period of time is to bring more blood to the affecte area. We will go along with the F. A. Book as heat would be easier for First Aiders to use, as long as you use ice first to prevent swelling.

CHAPTER VII

BURNS AND ILL EFFECTS OF HEAT AND COLD

Objective: *To relieve pain, prevent contamination, and treat for shock.*

Burns

Burns are a leading cause of accidental home deaths. In addition burns cause permanent disabilities, especially of the upper and lower extremities, and scarring. The economic costs are high because of the common need for prolonged hospitalization, close medical and nursing care, and restorative surgery of the face, hands, and other body parts. Wage loss may be high. Psychological effects may be far-reaching—especially when convalescence is long and distressing or when physical defects and scars remain.

Property damage from fire is enormous. About 300,000 homes are destroyed or damaged each year. The impact from loss of the home upon family members can seldom be fully appreciated except by actual experience.

Hazards associated with fire are (1) the searing and shock-producing effects of superheated air upon the lungs and respiratory passages, (2) the same effects of heat upon the skin, (3) the presence of carbon monoxide, (4) the absence of oxygen, (5) the effects of smoke in preventing escape, and (6) the hazard of jumping from buildings when trapped by fire.

There are three general kinds of burns: thermal burns, sunburn, and chemical burns.

Burns are also classified according to depth or degree:

First degree—the skin is reddened.

Second degree—blisters develop.

Third degree—there is deeper destruction, the underlying growth cells that continually form new skin being destroyed.

It is difficult or impossible to determine the degree of a burn at first. Often the degree differs in different parts of the affected area. Third-degree burns heal especially slowly. Since the growth cells are destroyed, new skin can grow only from the edges of the burn where such cells are still present.

Thermal burns

Prevention. Every homemaker should seek fire safety through determined, organized effort. Factors to consider include:

CONSTRUCTION AND EQUIPMENT. When building or buying a home, consider its fire safety in light of materials, arrangement, and fire-control features. Helpful information can be obtained from many sources. Install fire extinguishers in danger spots. Have a section of garden hose near a faucet for use in case of fire. Provide adequate guards for fireplaces, and insulation wherever a dangerous heating surface is near a wall or flammable material. In older homes, check the wiring lest it be defective or inadequate for

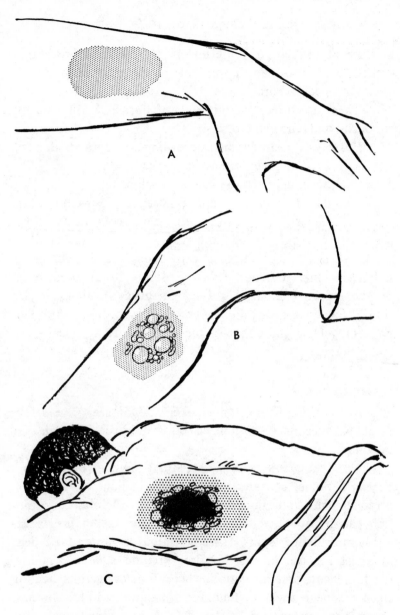

**Fig. 29   Degrees of burns.   A. First degree.   B. Second degree.
C. Third degree.**

large demands from many appliances, and check the heating system and electrical equipment for deterioration.

GOOD HOUSEKEEPING. Do not allow trash to accumulate anywhere in the house. It can cause spontaneous combustion. Use no flammable cleaning fluids. Hang clothes well away from stoves or fireplaces. See that curtains are not placed where they may blow into or near flames. Store flammable materials safely. Do not overload electric circuits. Take special precautions with small children. Never allow them to play around an open fire without supervision. Keep matches stored in a metal container, well out of their reach. Keep handles of pots turned away from the edge of the stove. Caution them about hot water faucets and never leave tubs of hot water where they can fall into them. Careless smoking habits are a common cause of home fires. Don't smoke in bed or when you are sleepy. Provide plenty of ash trays about the home.

EDUCATION. Have occasional home safety discussions concerning fire prevention, burn prevention, and what to do in case of fire. Home safety checks are a valuable feature of such education. Teach small children in such a way that morbid fears do not develop.

Escape from fire. Escape from fire is more likely if certain basic facts are understood. In case of fire, air near the floor is best because both heated air and carbon monoxide tend to rise. Fire travels faster when doors and windows are open. It is especially important to protect the respiratory passages, the hands, and the face. If any body part is covered with a thick textile, preferably wet, it is protected from heat for a time, but not against carbon monoxide.

Every family should have a plan for escape and additional action in case of home fire. The overriding objective is to escape. Beginning fires sometimes can be controlled by quick action, but there should be no delay in notifying the fire department. When attempting escape, open doors cautiously while crouching low and protected behind them because the next room may contain superheated air under pressure, a blast of which may be fatal when breathed. Jumping from upper stories is often fatal and unnecessary; rescue may be at hand. While awaiting rescue, close the doors and transoms, open the window slightly and breathe the incoming air. Attempts at rescue should not be foolhardy. It is difficult to locate people in a smoke-filled building and to find the way out quickly.

First aid. The objectives are to deal with or treat shock, relieve pain, and prevent contamination. The danger of infection is greatest in second and third degree burns. Burns often appear less deep at first than they are. Shock is a major hazard. It is commonly serious when the burn involves more than 10 percent of the body surface, and sometimes when the area is smaller. Most deaths occurring within the first few days are caused by shock. The patient with a serious burn should be immediately transported to a hospital.

The exclusion of air from a burn by the application of a thick dressing relieves pain and, if the dressing is sterile, prevents further contamination.

Obtain sterile dressings in sufficient quantity. If such are not available, treat clean cloths to render them as nearly sterile as possible by methods described in Chapter II. Dressings should be dry, because wet dressings stick more

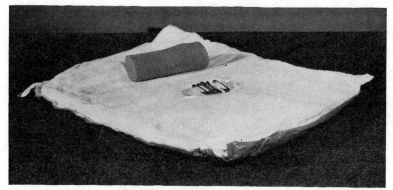

Fig. 30   Sterile burn pad.

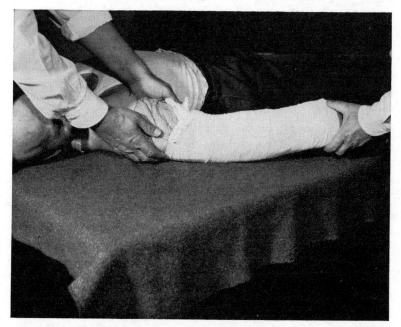

Fig. 31   Completed dressing of upper extremity using burn pad.

and allow germs to enter from the outside. It is usually best to cut the clothing off the burned areas rather than to unclothe the patient. Otherwise, simply protect and cover the burn and transport the patient. Apply the dressings in at least four layers, preferably six. Then add additional covering to exclude air still more, using clean, tightly woven material. Do not rupture blisters, although they may break through applying dressings. Be sure that your hands are thoroughly clean during the procedure.

If the burn is extensive, involving the trunk or a large part of an extremity, wrap a clean sheet or large towel around the part, cover additionally according to the weather, and transport the victim to a hospital.

For a burn of the eye, if pain can be tolerated, irrigate the eye gently to remove any foreign material. Cover with a dry sterile gauze pad or a dry, clean cloth, bandage, and *immediately* seek medical aid. Do not instill oil or ointments in the eye unless necessary to relieve pain pending medical care.

POSITION. How you position the patient depends upon the burned area. If the burn is of consequence, have the patient lie flat. Raise the foot of the bed or stretcher about 10 inches if the burn involves more than about 10 percent of the body. If the hand is burned, elevate it above the level of the body and keep it elevated. Patients with severe burns or burns of the lower extremities should be transported by stretcher.

FLUIDS. Severely burned patients need fluids, but fluids often cause nausea. Accordingly, judgment and observation are needed to administer fluids properly. If medical help will be available within twenty minutes or so, give fluids only to quench thirst. After this time is up and medical help has not arrived, begin giving at fifteen-minute intervals half-glass doses of a solution made by dissolving one-half level teaspoon table salt and one-half level teaspoon of baking soda in a quart of water.

Sunburn

Unlike thermal burns, sunburn is caused mainly by ultraviolet rays. A slight overexposure causes tiny blood vessels in the skin to dilate; the skin becomes red. As over-exposure increases, tissue injury starts, swelling of the skin occurs, blisters appear, and often fever and headache develop.

Prevention. Severe sunburn causes great discomfort and may require bed rest for many days. The most effective prevention lies in limiting the time of initial exposures. The first exposure should not be longer than ten to fifteen minutes. On sea and lake shores and at high altitudes, the increase of exposure time should be gradual; about one-third of the previous time if sunbaths are taken daily, and one-fourth or less if exposures are less frequent. Sunburn may follow exposure on a cloudy day.

Commercial preparations for protection against sunburn vary in their effects. Some have hardly any protecting effects; others are highly effective but may cause allergic reactions.

First aid. For mild sunburn, cold cream or such oils or greases as salad oil or shortening may relieve pain. Wash the hands before applying the material. Medicated creams may cause skin allergies. Butter or oleomargarine should not be applied.

A dressing should be used if blistering appears. Medical care is needed for extensive and severe cases. The injured area should not be exposed again to the sun until healing is completed.

Chemical burns

First aid for burns of the skin. When irritating chemicals come into contact with the skin or mucous membrane, injury usually commences instantly and first aid should be immediate. Among such chemicals are acids and alkalis, turpentine, some cleansing agents, lime and cement, petroleum products, some asphalt preparations, and some antiseptics. The essential first aid is to wash away the chemical completely with large quantities of water. If first aid directions against specific chemicals are available on labels or through industrial plant directions, follow them. In the absence of such directions, do not apply additional chemical, such as ammonia, to an acid burn. After removing the chemical, give additional first aid just as for any similar heat burn. These injuries, like all burns, should not be exposed to direct sunlight until healing has occurred.

First aid for burns of the eye. ACID BURNS. These are nonprogressive injuries. Wash the eye thoroughly with a solution of sodium bicarbonate (a teaspoonful of baking soda to a glass of water) or plain water. Have the patient close the eye, place an eye pad or a piece of cotton over the lid, and bandage. Seek *immediate* medical attention.

ALKALI BURNS. These are progressive injuries and an eye that at first appears to have slight surface injuries may develop deep inflammation and tissue destruction and be lost. Irrigate thoroughly with water, remove any particle of chemical, immobilize the lid with an eye pad or a piece of cotton over the skin surface, and *immediately* seek medical aid.

Ill Effects of Excessive Heat

Exposure to excessive heat may result in heat exhaustion, heat stroke, and heat cramps, the first-named being most common. In exhaustion cases, the temperature is approximately normal; in stroke, it is high. Most likely to be affected are the aged, the obese, the very young, alcohol addicts, and those suffering from any disease that impairs the strength of the entire body.

Prevention

Preventive measures relate to activity, clothing, fluids, possibly diet, and control of environment. Ill effects of heat are noted most often in northern sections. Persons living in tropical climates adapt their activity and clothing better to hot weather. The mid-day and early afternoon respite from activity is usual in tropical countries; exposure to direct sunlight is largely avoided, and light-colored clothing that reflects rather than absorbs sunlight is used. It would be wise if persons in northern climates followed these procedures during periods of intense heat.

Profuse perspiration helps cool the body, but it draws fluids and certain chemicals away. These must be replaced by intake of much water together with extra salt. The amounts needed vary with the amount of perspiration. A level teaspoonful of salt twice a day probably suffices for the chemical replacement in most working conditions, though under extreme conditions more may be required.

Formerly it was thought that one should avoid a heavy diet and partake only sparingly of proteins in hot weather. Now there is doubt that significant restriction of protein intake is necessary. It seems reasonable to avoid overeating. Hot weather and high humidity are especially likely to cause trouble to those doing heavy physical work. Control measures for indoors, such as adequate ventilation and wise air conditioning, are helpful to all, but particularly to workers exposed to high temperatures and humidity.

Heat exhaustion

This common condition may be mild or severe. In mild cases the patient feels unusually tired; he may have headache and nausea. In severe cases, perspiration is profuse, weakness extreme, the skin pale and clammy. The temperature is approximately normal. Vomiting may occur. Unconsciousness is rare.

First aid. Provide bed rest. Administer salt solution, a half teaspoonful per half-glass of water every fifteen minutes for three or four doses. These patients, though nauseated at first perhaps, usually can take the fluid after a period of bed rest. Medical care is needed for severe illness.

Heat stroke

Elderly people are prone to develop heat stroke. It may appear in them on hot days during such apparently mild activity as a walk. But they are not the only victims. The usual evidences are headache, dry skin, and rapid pulse. There may be dizziness and nausea. Unconsciousness occurs in many severe cases. The temperature is well above normal, often to 106, and sometimes above 109 degrees. Heat stroke is extremely dangerous. The toll is highest in the aged.

First aid. Medical care is urgently needed. The patient should be transported to a hospital as soon as possible. While awaiting such attention, bring the patient indoors, unclothe him, and provide bed rest. If he is conscious, give the salt solution, indicated as above, as tolerated. Sponge the body freely with alcohol or lukewarm water, to reduce the temperature to more tolerable levels, that is, 103 degrees or so. If a thermometer is not at hand, the only guides are the patient's general condition and his pulse rate. A rate below 110 per minute is probably associated with a tolerable temperature. Once this level is reached, caution is necessary. The temperature may decline more or it may rise again. Cease the sponging and observe the patient for ten minutes. If the temperature starts to rise again, renew the sponging cautiously. Give no stimulants; administer fluid and salt in small doses when full consciousness is evident. Later, provide covering according to his comfort.

Heat cramps

Cramps usually involve the abdominal muscles or the limbs. Loss of chemicals in profuse perspiration precedes the cramps. The condition may be associated with heat exhaustion.

First aid. Heat cramps usually respond better to firm pressure than to vigorous kneading. The application of

warm, wet towels also gives relief. In addition administer
salt water solution as described for heat exhaustion on page
80.

III Effects of Excessive Cold

Frostbite

Frostbite is produced by freezing of a part of the body.
Usually the frozen area is small, but occasionally it is extensive. The nose, ears, cheeks, fingers, and toes are affected
most often. People with poor circulation, such as the elderly and the exhausted, are not as resistant to cold as young
people. Intoxicated persons sometimes suffer extensive injury.

Prevention. Avoid undue exposure to cold when you
are exhausted or not well. Beware of high winds. Accept
the need to wear enough clothing, including an outer gar-
ment, perhaps of leather, to protect against the wind, an
extra pair of woolen socks, mittens rather than gloves, and
covering for the ears. If a part becomes cold, place it against
a warm body part or cover it more. Some physical activity,
including especially the frequent exercising of the fingers
and toes, is helpful. Avoid alcoholic drinks and smoking
immediately before and during exposure.

Symptoms. Just before frostbite occurs, the skin may
be slightly flushed. As frostbite develops, it changes to
white or greyish-yellow. Blisters may appear later. Pain
sometimes is felt early but subsides later. Often there is no
pain; the part feels intensely cold and numb. The victim
frequently is not aware of frostbite until someone tells him
or he observes the pale glossy skin.

First aid. Firm pressure against the part with the warm hand is helpful, but rubbing it with the hand or snow is definitely harmful. The experience of arctic explorers as well as military studies under cold weather conditions have shown that rubbing the injured tissue increases the risk of tissue death (gangrene).

Cover the frozen part with woolen material and provide extra clothing or blankets for the individual. Bring him indoors as soon as possible, give him a warm drink, and quickly re-warm the part if it is still cold and numb by immersing it in water at body temperature (90° F. to 100° F.) *but not hot* water, or by gently wrapping it in warm

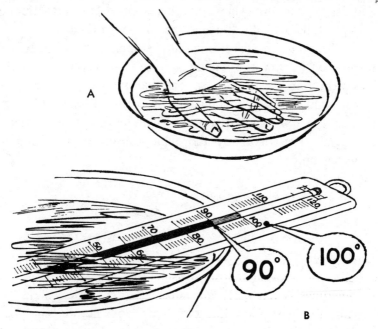

Fig. 32 A. One example of warming frostbite. B. Water should be within these ranges.

blankets. Handle the frozen part with the greatest care. Do not apply hot water bottles or heat lamps, nor place the frozen part near a hot stove, because excessive heat may increase the damage. Once the part is re-warmed, encourage the patient to exercise injured fingers and toes. Do not disturb blisters. If essential travel must be undertaken, apply a sterile dressing that widely overlaps the injury before putting on shoes or mittens.

Prolonged exposure to cold

Symptoms. When a person is exposed to excessive cold for a long time, he becomes numb, movement is difficult, and irresistible drowsiness overtakes him. He staggers, his eyesight fails, he falls and may become unconscious.

First aid. If breathing has stopped, begin artificial respiration. Bring the victim into a warm room quickly. Re-warm him as rapidly as possible by wrapping him in warm blankets or by placing him in a tub of warm (78° F. to 82° F.) *but not hot* water. When he reacts, give him a hot drink. Dry the body thoroughly if water was used to re-warm him.

CHAPTER VIII

COMMON EMERGENCIES—PART ONE

Heart Attack

About nine million people in this country have heart disease; a far greater number have changes occurring in their bodies that may lead to heart trouble. The disease is fairly common in young people because of congenital defects, as a result of rheumatic fever, or less often as a result of high blood pressure or toxic disease. Heart failure or attack is far more common in persons middle-aged or older, sometimes as a holdover but more often because of hardening of the heart arteries or as a result of high blood pressure.

Symptoms. Symptoms include shortness of breath, chest pain, bluish color of the lips and about the finger nails, a chronic cough, and swelling of the ankles. Other disorders may cause the same symptoms, which call for prompt medical attention.

In addition to the chronic complaints listed above, there may be acute attacks, presenting two principal symptoms: (1) extreme shortness of breath and (2) pain. These symptoms may occur in combination, but usually one or the other is outstanding.

Heart disease usually develops gradually. The evidences appear in mild form first and become more severe or frequent if the disease progresses. In the cases with gradually developing symptoms, the patient ordinarily seeks medical attention and learns what to do in case of an acute attack. Thus, the first aider's responsibility is to assist in getting medical care. Often, however, an acute heart attack is the first inkling to the patient of his trouble. In such unheralded attacks, pain over the heart or down the arms may be the outstanding evidence of heart trouble.

The pain is located most often in the chest, particularly under the sternum, or breastbone, and sometimes spreads down the left arm or into the head and neck and occasionally elsewhere. Sometimes the pain in the arm and shoulder is severe, and the chest pain may be minimal. First aiders should be aware that pain in the upper abdomen, especially in people of middle age or older, frequently reflects an acute heart attack that urgently requires medical attention. Indigestion manifested by nausea and vomiting is often associated with heart attacks. The symptoms may be attributed wrongly to stomach or gall bladder disease.

The pain in the chest or upper abdomen may be so severe as to induce profuse perspiration and to cause the patient to walk about rather than lie flat. In one type of attack, the patient insists upon lying absolutely still in a position of choice; such attacks commonly subside within a few minutes.

Attacks with milder pain do occur. They should not be dismissed lightly. The degree of pain is not an accurate index of severity of the underlying condition.

Prevention. Perhaps the most important measure is to have a checkup each year after the age of forty. The prevention of heart disease relates to a way of life as well as to special measures.

Control of weight is of cardinal importance. There is evidence that emotional tension contributes indirectly and directly to heart trouble. It is probable that a midday siesta of twenty minutes or more, bringing relaxation from the responsibilities of the day, is worthwhile. Strenuous exercise should not be attempted by persons unaccustomed to it, the danger being greater as they become older.

First aid. If the patient has been under medical care, the first aider should assist in administering prescribed medicine and in carrying out other measures advised by the physician.

If medical care has not been given previously, advice should be obtained at once, meanwhile deferring transportation.

For faintness, the lying-down position is best, usually without a pillow, although the comfort of the patient is a good guide. Raising the legs may be helpful.

For shortness of breath, raise the head and chest to a position most comfortable by providing as many pillows as needed. Provide adequate ventilation, guarding against drafts and cold.

When pain is acute, the lying-down position again is best but the pain may not permit such position at first. You can inform the patient that this position demands less strain than the upright. Do so without alarming him. In many cases of acute pain, the patient has a sense of impending death. He benefits from encouraging words, from tactful suggestions, from knowledge that medical help is forthcoming. It is best not to show extreme concern and to avoid reference to the attack as being a heart attack. Medication should be given only under the direction of a physician.

In most cases the patient should be hospitalized where he can be given oxygen, if necessary, and other medication. However, transportation throws some added strain upon him and should not be attempted until medical advice is obtained, if this is possible within a reasonable time. If transportation is finally attempted, the patient should not be disturbed during the planning, nor subjected first to such ordeals as changing his clothes, shaving, and bathing. It is extremely important that he remain recumbent during transportation. If he is out of doors, use a stretcher or cot.

Apoplexy (stroke)

Apoplexy is usually caused by a blood clot or hemorrhage involving a vessel of the brain. The most common underlying factors are hardening of the arteries and high blood pressure. The preventive measures against heart disease apply in general also against this disorder.

Symptoms. The evidences vary according to the severity and location of the damage to the brain. In case of extensive brain damage, there is unconsciousness, heavy breathing, and paralysis of the upper or lower extremity, or both, on one side of the body. In the unconscious person, the paralysis can be detected by the fact that the extremity is not moved by the patient and by a looseness or a lack of muscle tension when the extremity is raised slightly. The pupils of the eyes may be unequal in size.

If the damage to the brain is slight, the nature of the

episode may not be recognized. There may be dizziness or headache, a sudden partial failure of memory, change of disposition, muscular difficulty involving some body part, a speech defect, or ringing in the ears. When any of these symptoms appear suddenly in older persons, a "small stroke" perhaps is the cause. Not infrequently the evidence is noted when the patient awakes in the morning.

First aid. For the severe attack, with a comatose or semi-comatose patient, keep the patient flat. If the patient is having difficulty breathing, he should be turned on his side to allow secretions to drool from the mouth. Provide moderate covering. Do not give any fluids or food until medical care has started unless an unusually long interval is going to elapse before the patient can be seen by a physician.

Medical care obviously is needed immediately.

The first aider should be alert to the possibility of small strokes as described above. His only procedure then is to suggest medical attention, meanwhile providing protection of the patient against accident or physical exertion. Do not use heat.

Simple Fainting

Simple fainting is a reaction of the nervous system that results in a temporary diminution of the blood supply to the brain. Fear, bad news, (good news sometimes, too), the viewing of an injury or blood, and the prospect of a medical treatment are among many precipitating causes. If one is not feeling well, is tired, worried, or obliged to stand quietly in a stuffy room, he is more susceptible to fainting.

Prevention. Have the person lie flat with the head low if he feels faint. This is the best procedure. If it is not feasible at the moment, have him lower his head between the knees and breathe deeply.

First aid. Put the patient on his back and keep him recumbent until recovery is complete, for perhaps ten minutes or more. Otherwise he may faint again when he gets up. It has been a common custom to apply a whiff from an ammonia ampule or bottle to the person's nostrils. This does no harm; the nervous system is jolted slightly, possibly a recurrence of fainting soon after is somewhat less likely, and the procedure gives both the patient and the helper the pleasant feeling that something special has been done.

The person who has fainted will recover consciousness almost immediately upon reaching the recumbent position. If he fails to do so, medical advice should be sought because the case is not simple fainting. If fainting occurs frequently, consult a physician.

Epileptic Convulsions

Epilepsy is not a specific disease but rather a symptom-complex based upon many causes. Among these are injury and infection. During recent years, research has extended greatly the medical understanding about epilepsy and has made available more effective treatment. The untreated patients and occasionally some of those under care are subject to attacks of unconsciousness. These may last only a second or so and perhaps be unrecognized; or they may be obvious, associated with a fall and with convulsions involving the entire body. The violent attack usually subsides within a few minutes or less, but the person may suffer injury during the convulsions by striking against objects or by biting his tongue. When known epileptics suspect an attack, they should seek a quiet place immediately and lie down with a bit between the teeth.

First aid. Do not restrain the person in his convulsions, but protect him against injury. Push away nearby objects. Try gently to prevent him from biting the tongue by placing an appropriate object, such as the edge of a book cover or spoon handle wrapped in a clean handkerchief or napkin, between his upper and lower teeth on one side of the mouth. Do not obstruct breathing. When the jerking is over, loosen the clothing about the neck and allow him to lie flat with the head turned to one side.

When he regains consciousness, do not question him or disturb him. These patients are understandably sensitive. Try in all ways to guard them against embarrassment. Patients usually are drowsy after the episode and need a period of undisturbed sleep. If they arise immediately and walk about, they may have another attack. Therefore, provide for undisturbed rest. Prevent aspiration of vomitus into the lungs by turning the head to one side or by having the patient lie on his abdomen.

Unconsciouness—Cause Unknown

Asphyxia, deep shock, poisoning (especially by sleep-producing drugs), head injury, heat stroke, heart attack, apoplexy, and epilepsy have already been discussed as causes of unconsciousness, and first aid measures have been suggested. It is possible that you may encounter an unconscious person, the nature of whose trouble is unknown. In such event, you can readily classify the person as belonging to one of two groups: (1) Cases requiring artificial respiration, and (2) cases where breathing is adequate.

If the person is not breathing or has extreme difficulty in breathing he would be in the first group, provided circumstances suggest that artificial respiration would be helpful, as with the possibility of gas, barbiturate, and alcohol poisoning or electric shock, for example. First aiders should not give artificial respiration invariably when they find a person unconscious, but only when the patient is obviously not breathing adequately.

The first aider should search the patient's effects for a statement that he is a diabetic taking insulin (p. 169).

First aid. Administer artificial respiration promptly if required and carry out the other first aid measures as described in the chapter on artificial respiration. Turn the head to the side and place the patient on his abdomen to enable him to breathe better and to prevent aspiration of vomitus.

In either group, notify a physician and, if indicated, a police officer. Do not disturb the victim, the personal belongings, or any other possible evidence if crime, accident, or suicide may be considered, except as essential to save the person's life.

Since you do not know the nature and location of the trouble, consider that any body part may be affected. Keep all parts immobile and use a stretcher or cot for transportation if that must be undertaken.

Foreign Body in the Eye

If there is a foreign body in the eye, do not rub the eye. The most common place for foreign bodies to lodge is on the inner surface of the upper lid. Tell the patient to look down. Grasp the edge of the upper lid moderately firmly, make slight pressure on the skin surface of the lid with the side of a blunt pencil or the side of a match stick, and try to turn the inner surface of the lid outward. If the

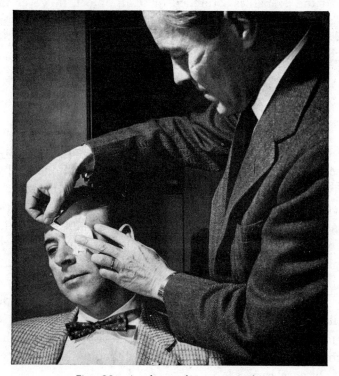

Fig. 33 Applying the eye patch.

foreign body is seen on the inner surface of the lid, it can easily be removed by touching it with the corner of a clean handkerchief. If the foreign body is seen on the surface of the cornea (the clear front part of the eye), have the patient wink several times and see if it can be dislodged. If the foreign body is embedded and cannot be dislodged, do not attempt to remove it. Have the patient close the eye, place a pad or a piece of moist cotton over the closed lid, bandage, and obtain medical attention.

If the eyeball is scratched or if an object, however tiny, penetrates the eyeball even a small fraction of an inch, it is urgent that medical care be obtained at once. The injury may be extremely serious though it appears minor. If protection is needed meanwhile, apply a loose bandage.

Foreign Body in the Throat or Air Passages

If a foreign body lodges in the throat or air passages, violent choking commonly results. Sometimes the object descends into the lungs. If so, it cannot be eliminated by a normal process. If it remains in the lungs, it will cause an infection unless removed by bronchoscope or operation. Occasionally, a choking incident is absent or mild; but if the object remains in the air passages or lungs, a chronic cough or an infection develops soon, or less often, after several weeks. The commonest objects are food items— nuts, seeds, and shells; others are small hardware items, pins, needles, dental items, bones, jewelry, coins, and toys. The victims most often are children, but older people may have trouble because of loose dentures, difficulty in masticating food, or carelessness.

Prevention. More children die from this mishap than

from any childhood communicable disease except polio-myelitis and meningitis. Small children should not be given such foods as peanuts, popcorn, and cake containing nuts before they have their first teeth and have learned to masti-cate well. Meat should be finely chopped for small chil-dren. They should not be permitted to run about while eating. Small objects should not be left within reach of small children. Many cases of aspiration of foreign bodies in adults and children result from careless food preparation and from hurried and careless eating. The habit of placing pins, needles, nails, and the like in the mouth endangers the adult who does it and sets a bad example for the child.

First aid.

1. Let the patient attempt to cough up the ob-ject. Do *not* probe with the fingers into the throat lest you push the object farther down. Probing contributes no more than the cough-ing will. If the victim is a child, turn him upside down and smack him on the back be-tween the shoulder blades.
2. Do not distract the patient from his attempt to cough and breathe effectively by showing your alarm or by asking him questions.
3. Always take him to a physician or the nearest hospital emergency ward, unless the object is expelled, even though symptoms subside.
4. If breathing ceases (rare), give artificial respiration and try to clear the airway with fingers or forceps. Life-saving in cases of this type may be exceedingly urgent.

Foreign Body in the Food Passages

If foreign objects are swallowed, they most often pass harmlessly along and are excreted. Bobby pins and open safety pins are passed along the digestive tract in many cases. Nevertheless, there is definite danger that the object may become lodged or may have entered the air passages instead. Bones most often cause trouble in the food passages, requiring surgical intervention, that is, use of an extractor instrument or an operation. Other objects sometimes requiring extraction include coins and discs, food, pins, buttons, shells, and toys. Preventive measures are the same as against foreign objects in the air passages. Persons should take care when eating food containing bones and remember not to talk while foreign objects are in the mouth. Symptoms from swallowed objects may be absent early unless the object lodges in the esophagus, when pain, difficulty in swallowing, or a feeling of lodgment are usually present.

First aid. Take the patient to the physician. Even though symptoms are absent, the object may be lodged in the food passage or perhaps in the air passage.

Drive safely while transporting the patient to the medical facility, though the distance may be many miles. The situation is not one of extreme urgency in case of swallowed objects. Remain calm, thus guarding the patient against fears created by excitement and hysteria.

If feeding is necessary—in the case of small children or because of long delay in getting medical attention, provide the usual diet. Do not give cathartics or bulky foods.

CHAPTER IX

TRANSPORTATION

Objective *To avoid subjecting the patient to unnecessary disturbance during planning, preparation, and transfer; to prevent injured body parts from twisting, bending, and shaking.*

The most common first aid procedure associated with serious accidents and illness is transportation. It often is one of the most time-consuming procedures. Perhaps more harm is done through improper transportation than through any other measure associated with emergency assistance. The harm springs from lack of planning, from lack of preparation or improper preparation of the patient for transportation, and from use of poorly adapted methods; therefore, take the necessary time and effort to provide good transportation.

Sometimes the first aider is under emotional pressure when he deals with an accident victim. Perhaps he has never encountered a serious accident before. He may know that head injury cases and those with fractures and internal injuries usually benefit from a period of rest before trans-

[97]

portation. But when the responsibility for first aid is his and he notes the bad condition of the patient, he may fall before the pressure of the situation and give hurried transportation by improper means. It requires calmness to seek a stretcher or cot and a suitable vehicle in case of a highway accident, particularly if the nearest home is a half mile away, the victim is in serious condition, and the weather is inclement. But the time for good transportation is precisely when the victim is in bad condition.

Methods of Transfer

These include special methods for short-distance transfers, the walking assist, manual carries, transfer by supporting devices such as stretchers and cots, and transfer by vehicles.

It is difficult for inexperienced people to lift and carry a person gently. Their efforts may not be well coordinated. They need careful explanations. It is wise to practice the procedure first, using a practice subject. In all cases, anyone who helps carry a patient should guard against losing his balance, a mishap of surprising frequency, even when three or more carriers are used. The carriers should lift gradually and with proper technique, so that they do not suffer back injury.

The short-distance transfer

This refers to such procedures as removing a victim from a wrecked automobile, from a place of danger, public scrutiny, or inclement weather and carrying him to or from a vehicle or bed. The procedure may cause additional injury

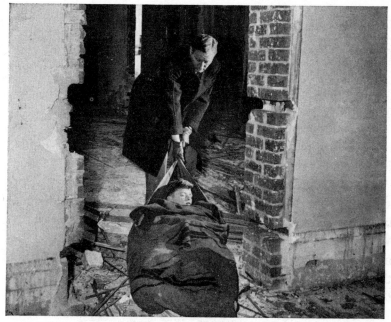

Fig. 34 The blanket drag.

to the victim, because it must be done sometimes before a checkup to locate the injured parts can be made or because injured parts have not been immobilized. Obviously, before a short transfer is attempted, a check for injuries should be made and if possible injured parts should be immobilized.

Pulling the victim to safety. If the victim must be pulled to safety, he should be pulled in the direction of the long axis of his body, not sideways. The danger is less if a blanket or similar object can be placed beneath him, so that he can ride the blanket.

Lifting the victim to safety. If a person must be lifted to safety before a check for injuries can be made, the carriers should try to protect all parts of the body from the tensions of lifting. The body should not be jackknifed (lifted by head and heels only). An attempt should be made to give adequate support to each extremity, the head, and the back, keeping the entire body in a straight line and maintaining it immobile.

Sometimes, although a checkup can be made, immobilization of an injured part, such as an extremity, is not feasible until the patient is moved a short distance. Such a situation should be rare. If it is encountered, the first aider should devote himself to the injured extremity, placing one hand just above the injured area and one just below it. While helpers lift the body and another helper lifts the main weight of the injured extremity, the first aider keeps the immediate area of the injury from bending and twisting.

The best device for short-distance transfers is the stretcher or cot. Improvisations can be made from blankets or similar items together with two sturdy poles. Patients can be transported comfortably for long distances over rough terrain on cots or stretchers.

It is important to remember that the short-distance transfer is harmful unless the injured parts are immobilized. "Splint them where they lie" unless there is urgent danger in delay.

The vehicle transfer

Unless there is unusual urgency it is best to wait until an ambulance is available. Some trucks give a smooth ride; others do not. A few automobiles have space for a stretcher, though the arrangement may not permit constant observation of the patient. Aside from rare exceptions, the drive should be at moderate speeds, with gentle stops and starts, and with observation of all safety rules. However well-splinted or otherwise immobilized an injured part may be, the fracture or injured area sustains some harmful effect from constant swaying and jolting of the vehicle as it rounds turns, slows down, increases speed, or encounters dips and elevations.

Planning for Transportation

This should be done with responsible relatives or friends. Occasionally, the victim must be consulted. Once the decision to transport is made, the means and method must be planned. What vehicle will be used? How will it be obtained? What steps must be taken to prepare the patient? What supporting device, such as stretcher, cot, or mattress, is needed? Exactly what shall be the function of each assistant?

Preparation of the Patient

Preliminary first aid measures may be required for accident victims. Often they benefit from a period of rest before transfer. If the subject is ill rather than injured, the first aider customarily has no special patient-preparation responsibilities unless delegated by the physician. Too often the patient is subjected to disturbing and exhausting preparation before transportation is begun.

It is most important to remember that people who may have head injuries, fractures of such bones as those of the thigh, leg, arm, and pelvis, or possible back injuries should not be transported sitting up in passenger automobiles. The injured parts need immobilization; the body should be recumbent on a comfortable support; the patient should be transported with safety.

CHAPTER X

FIRST AID SKILLS
FOR
STANDARD COURSE

Anchoring a Bandage

1. Place the end of the bandage on a bias at the starting point.
2. Encircle the part, allowing the corner of the bandage end to protrude.
3. Turn down the protruding tip of the bandage and encircle the part again.

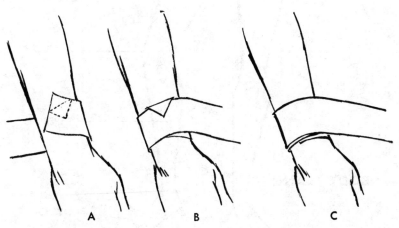

Fig. 35 Anchoring a bandage. A. First step. B. Second Step. C. Third step.

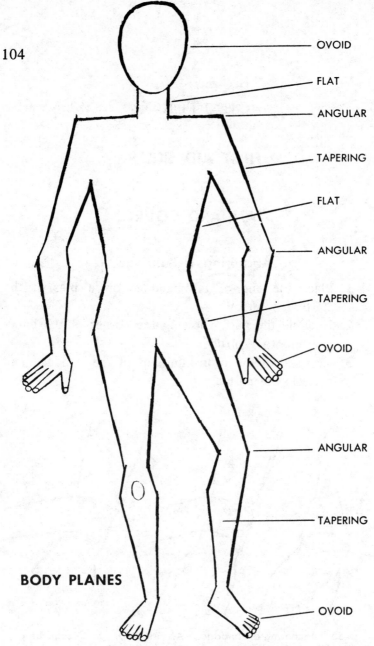

104

OVOID

FLAT

ANGULAR

TAPERING

FLAT

ANGULAR

TAPERING

OVOID

ANGULAR

TAPERING

OVOID

BODY PLANES

Fig. 36   The body planes.

The Circular Turn

Circular turns simply encircle the part with each layer of bandage superimposed on the previous one. It is the simplest of all bandage turns. However, its use is limited to covering parts of uniform width, such as the toe, neck, and head.

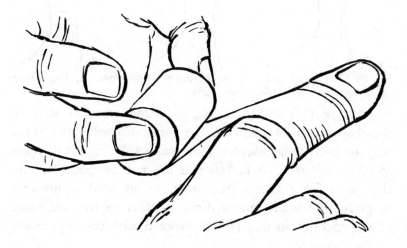

Fig. 37 The circular turn.

Spiral Turns

Spiral turns are those directed obliquely to the long axis of the part. They are called "closed" spiral turns if each turn of bandage overlaps *one-third* to *one-half* the width of the preceding one. There should be no visible areas of skin or dressing between the turns of a closed spiral bandage. Open or coarse spiral turns are oblique turns with a greater measure of obliqueness than closed spiral turns; no turn

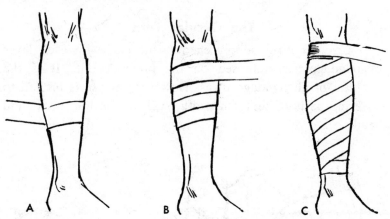

Fig. 38 The spiral turn. A. Anchoring the bandage. B. The closed spiral turn.   C. The open spiral turn.

overlaps part of the preceding one, and areas of skin or dressing are visible between the turns. Closed spiral turns may be used to bandage a part that varies in width; open spiral turns are used to retain a dressing temporarily, one that must be changed frequently, or to hold a dressing in place with a few initial turns in order to free the hand of the operator so that he can proceed with the application of the bandage.

Figure-of-Eight Turns

The figure-of-eight turn consists basically of two spiral loops of bandage, one up and one down, crossing each other thus forming an 8. It can be used to bandage an entire limb or a joint.

Recurrent Turns

Recurrent turns of bandage are those that wind back and forth over a part and are not in themselves capable of retaining a dressing in position. They must be fastened

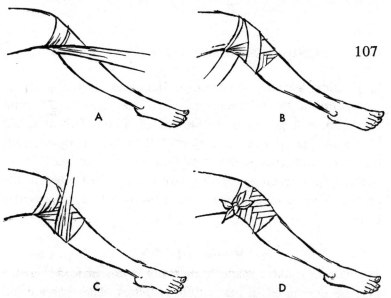

Fig. 39 The figure-of-eight turn. A. Anchoring the bandage. B. Covering the injured area. C. Completing the figure-of-eight turn. D. The finished bandage.

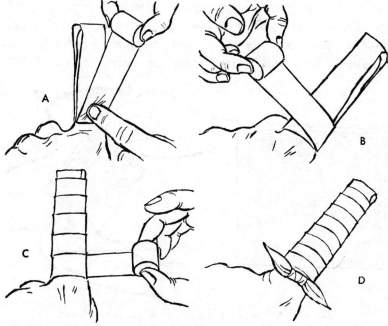

Fig. 40 The recurrent turn. A. Start of recurrent turn. B. Circular turn holds recurrent turns. C. Circular turn continued. D. Finished bandage.

in position by circular turns of bandages at the folds of the recurrent turns. Recurrent turns are used in covering the scalp, a finger, and the stumps of limbs. The first fold is usually placed over one side of the part being covered; the next fold covers the opposite side of the part being covered, and each succeeding fold is worked toward the center. The recurrent turns are held in place by circular turns.

Gauze Squares

Gauze squares made from many layers of folded gauze may be purchased in many different sizes. These are sealed in individual packages, which ensure sterility, at least for a time, if they are unbroken. Special care should be taken when removing the gauze square from the envelope and placing it over the wound. Tear one corner of the envelope, take a small corner of the dressing between the thumb and forefinger and pull it free from the envelope. *DO NOT*

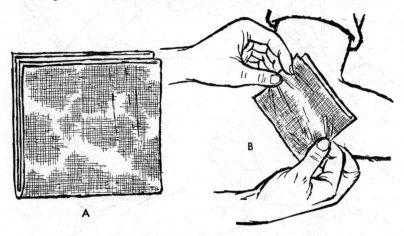

Fig 41   A. Gauze square.   B. Applied to elbow.

touch or breathe on the side to be placed over the wound. After the dressing is placed over the wound, it may be held in place with the hand until it is secured by a bandage.

Adhesive Compress

Adhesive gauze compresses usually consist of a 1-inch pad of sterile gauze placed in the middle of a 1-inch by 3-inch strip of adhesive. This is usually covered with one

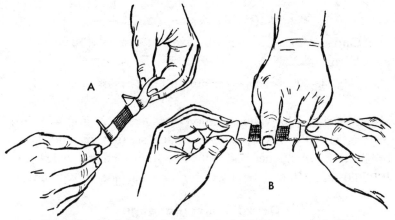

Fig. 42   A. Adhesive compress.   B. Compress applied.

layer of crinoline to protect the adhesive. These compresses are available in sizes up to 6 inches wide; the desired width may be cut off as needed. This form of compress is not as easy to keep sterile as the individually packed smaller sizes. The adhesive compress acts as both a dressing and a bandage for small cuts or scratches.

Bandage Compress

The bandage compress consists of a pad made of several thicknesses of sterile gauze sewed to the middle of a strip

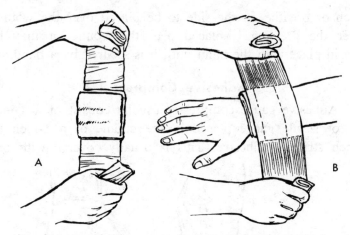

Fig. 43   A. Bandage compress.   B. Compress applied.

of gauze or muslin. The common sizes are 2, 3, and 4 inches square. Usually this dressing is made so that by cutting or breaking a stitch the pad may be unfolded to twice the original size. It can be used for any surface it will cover.

Gauze Roller Bandage

Gauze roller bandages are made of strips of sterilized cotton gauze in tight rolls. Common widths are 1, 2, and 3 inches and the length is usually 10 yards. The roller bandage is well adapted for use on the extremities because it can be applied neatly and snugly on the irregular surfaces of these parts. Care must be taken so that the bandage is not applied so tight as to impede circulation. Adhesive tape is used to hold the bandage in place. If tape is not available, tear or cut the end far enough to encircle the part, tie a single knot to prevent further splitting, then carry the ends around the part in opposite directions and tie.

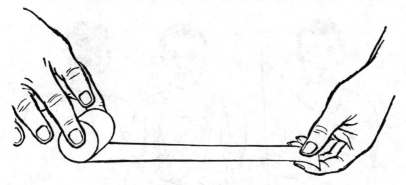

Fig. 44 The gauze roller bandage.

Plain Strips of Cloth

Plain strips of cloth are used as substitutes for gauze roller bandages. These substitutes are *not* medically sterile and should not come in direct contact with the wound. These strips of cloth may be torn from a sheet or yard goods in any desired width and length, then rolled. They are applied in the same manner as the roller bandage.

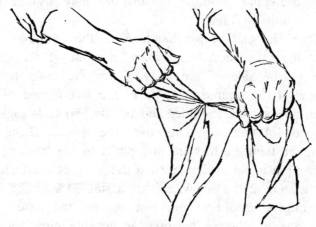

Fig. 45 Substitute for gauze roller bandage.

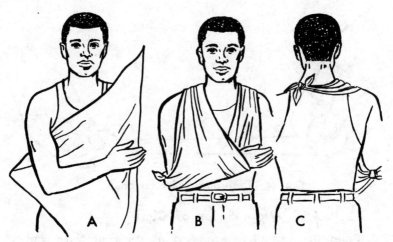

Fig: 46   The arm sling. A. Step one.   B. Step two.   C. Step three.

Arm Sling

Prepare a triangular piece of cloth approximately 55 inches across the base and 36-40 inches along the sides. Regular triangular bandages of this size may also be purchased in unit packages.

Place one end of the bandage on the uninjured side and let the other end hang down in front of the chest, parallel to the side of the body. Carry the point behind the elbow of the injured arm. Carry the second end of the bandage up over the shoulder and tie the two ends together at the side of the neck (not over the spine). Bring the point of the bandage forward and pin it to the front of the sling. If a pin is not available, twist the point of the bandage until it is snug at the elbow, and tie a single knot. The ends of the fingers should extend just beyond the base. This permits one to observe whether or not the circulation is cut off.

In all cases of injury to the hand or lower forearm, the sling should be adjusted so that the hand is elevated 4 or 5 inches above the level of the elbow.

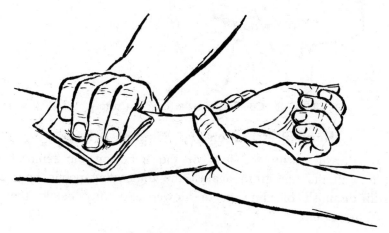

Fig. 47   Direct pressure over wound.

Direct Pressure

The first step in controlling bleeding is *direct pressure* over the wound area. You can do this best by placing the cleanest material available (sterile gauze is best) against the bleeding point and applying firm pressure with your hand until a bandage can be applied. If the part can be elevated, it will aid the control of bleeding. Most wounds can be cared for in this manner.

Finger Pressure on Brachial Artery

Pressure on the brachial artery against the underlying bone will diminish the flow of blood to the upper extremity below the pressure point.

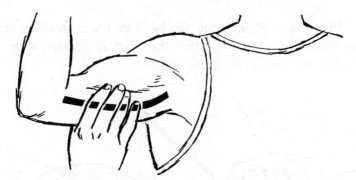

Fig. 48   Compressing the brachial artery.

Hand Pressure on the Femoral Artery

Pressure with the heel of the hand on the femoral artery in the mid-groin against the underlying pelvic bone will diminish bleeding in the lower extremity below the pressure point.

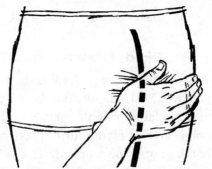

Fig. 49   Compressing the femoral artery.

The Tourniquet

Use of the tourniquet

The tourniquet is mentioned principally to discourage its use. Its application may cause tissue injury; it may completely shut off the entire blood supply to the part below, and the pressure device itself often cuts into or injures the skin. It is used far too often. THE TOURNIQUET SHOULD BE USED ONLY FOR SEVERE, LIFE-THREATENING HEMORRHAGE THAT CANNOT BE CONTROLLED BY OTHER MEANS. It is only rarely required. Tourniquets should be used only when severe bleeding involves an extremity in which large arteries are severed, or in cases of partial or complete severance of a body part. These are the only instances where application of a tourniquet may be justified. The procedure for application is as follows:

1. Place the tourniquet close above the wound, between the body and the wound, but not at the wound edge. There should be normal skin between the tourniquet and the wound. If the wound is near a joint, the application should be made at the nearest practical point above the joint.

2. Make sure that it is applied tightly enough to stop bleeding. Improperly applied, especially if not tight enough, it may increase venous bleeding and hasten death.

3. Once the tourniquet is applied, the patient should be taken as soon as possible to a physician. The release of the tourniquet, when once applied, should be carried out only by a physician or by medical personnel prepared to control hemorrhage and replace blood volume adequately. Experience has shown that a properly applied tourniquet can be left in place for one or two hours without causing further damage to the extremity.

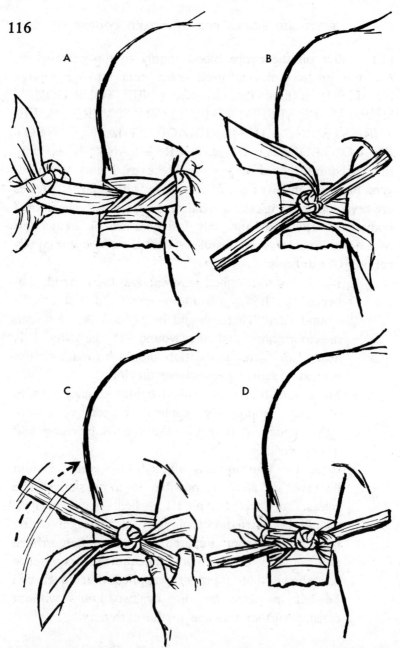

Fig. 50 Application of tourniquet. A. Wrap twice around arm, tie half-knot. B. Place "windlass" over half-knot. C. Finish knot and turn windlass to tighten. D. Secure windlass with tails of tourniquet.

4. A notation should always be made and attached to the victim, giving the location and the hour of application of the tourniquet.
5. Improvised tourniquets should be made of flat material about two inches wide (a cravat bandage, stockings, or a belt, for example). Try to avoid using rope, wire, or sash cord; they may cause injuries to the underlying tissues and blood vessels.

Application of the tourniquet

1. Wrap the material tightly *twice* around the limb if possible and tie a half knot.
2. Place a short stout stick or similar article on the half knot and tie a full knot.
3. Twist the stick to tighten the tourniquet until the flow of blood ceases.
4. Secure the stick in place with the loose end of the tourniquet, another strip of cloth, or other improvised material.

A Technique for Administering Manual Artificial Respiration

There are various effective ways to give artificial respiration manually, each with its advantages and disadvantages. The *back pressure-arm lift method* is recommended as best for general use. The standard technique is as follows:

1. *Position of the subject.* Place the subject in the face-down, prone position. Bend his elbows and place the hands one upon the other. Turn his face

slightly to one side, placing the cheek upon his hands. Always be sure the tongue does not block the air passage.

2. *Position of the operator.* Kneel on either the right or left knee at the head of the subject facing him. Place the knee at the side of the subject's head close to the forearm. Place the opposite foot near the elbow. If it is more comfortable, kneel on both knees, one on either side of the subject's head. Place your hands upon the flat of the subject's back in such a way that the palms lie just below an imaginary line running between the armpits. With the tips of the thumbs just touching, spread the fingers downward and outward.

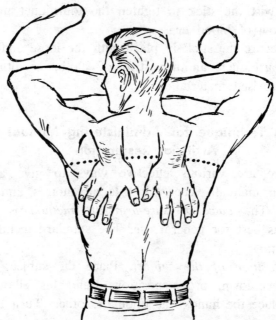

Fig. 51.1 Position of the subject.

3. *Compression phase.* Rock forward until the arms are approximately vertical and allow the weight of the upper part of your body to exert slow, steady, even pressure downward upon the hands. This forces air out of the lungs. Your elbows should be kept straight and the pressure exerted almost directly downward on the back.

4. *Position for expansion phase.* Release the pressure, avoiding a final thrust, and commence to rock slowly backward. Place your hands upon the subject's arms just above his elbows.

5. *Expansion phase.* Draw his arms upward and toward you. Apply just enough lift to feel re-

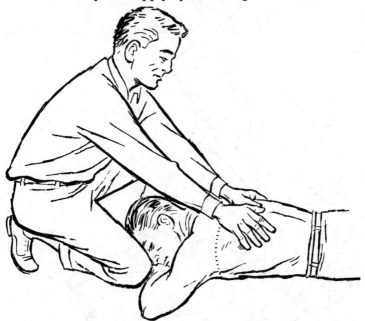

Fig. 51.2 Position of the operator.

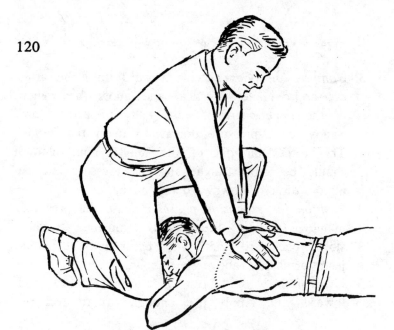

Fig. 51.3   Compression phase.

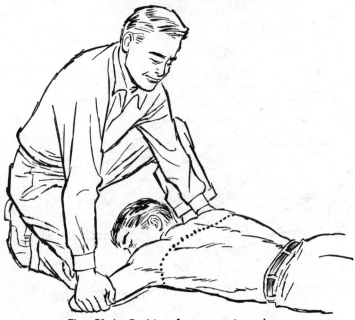

Fig. 51.4   Position for expansion phase.

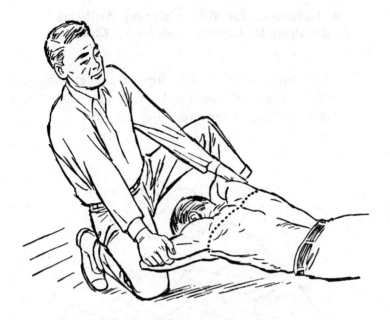

Fig. 51.5 Expansion phase.

sistance and tension at the subject's shoulders. Do not bend your elbows, and as you rock backward the subject's arms will be drawn toward you. Then lower the arms to the ground. This completes the full cycle. The arm lift expands the chest by pulling on the chest muscles, arching the back, and relieving the weight on the chest.

The cycle should be repeated 12 times per minute at a steady rate. The compression and expansion phases should occupy about equal time, with the release periods being of minimum duration.

A Technique for Administering Artificial Respiration to Infants and Small Children

1. Clear the mouth of any foreign matter with the middle finger of one hand. With the same finger press the tongue forward. (Fig. 52.1)

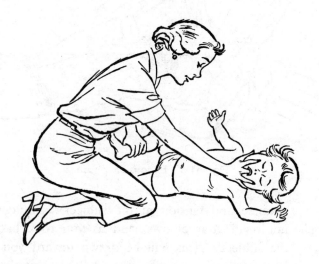

Fig. 52.1

2. Now place the child in a face-down, head-down position and pat him firmly on the back with the free hand. This should help dislodge any foreign object in the air passage. (Fig. 52.2)

ILLUSTRATIVE COLOR PLATES

- The Circulatory System
- The Skeletal System
- The Musculature
- The Internal Organs
- Poisonous Snakes
- Poisonous Plants

THE CIRCULATORY SYSTEM

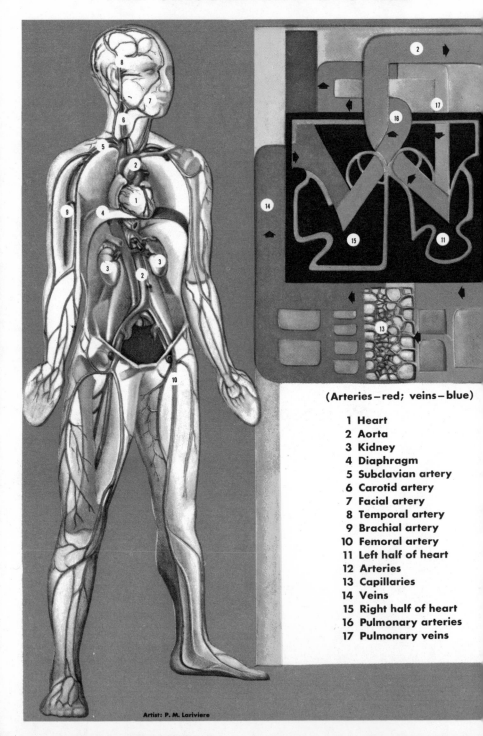

(Arteries—red; veins—blue)

1 Heart
2 Aorta
3 Kidney
4 Diaphragm
5 Subclavian artery
6 Carotid artery
7 Facial artery
8 Temporal artery
9 Brachial artery
10 Femoral artery
11 Left half of heart
12 Arteries
13 Capillaries
14 Veins
15 Right half of heart
16 Pulmonary arteries
17 Pulmonary veins

Artist: P. M. Lariviere

THE SKELETON

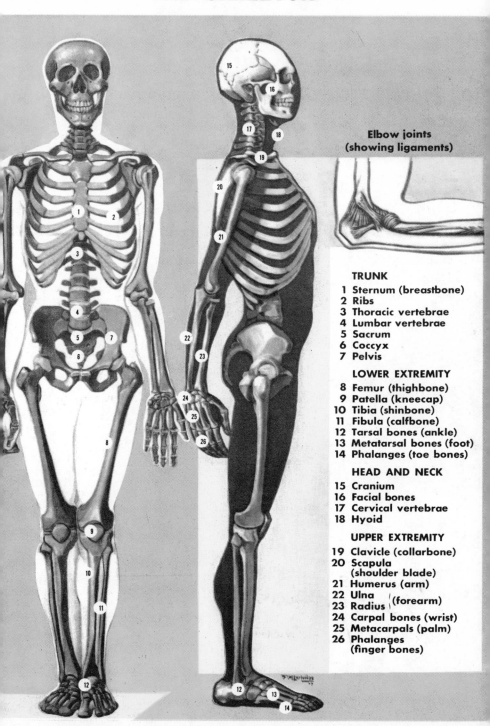

Elbow joints
(showing ligaments)

TRUNK
1 Sternum (breastbone)
2 Ribs
3 Thoracic vertebrae
4 Lumbar vertebrae
5 Sacrum
6 Coccyx
7 Pelvis

LOWER EXTREMITY
8 Femur (thighbone)
9 Patella (kneecap)
10 Tibia (shinbone)
11 Fibula (calfbone)
12 Tarsal bones (ankle)
13 Metatarsal bones (foot)
14 Phalanges (toe bones)

HEAD AND NECK
15 Cranium
16 Facial bones
17 Cervical vertebrae
18 Hyoid

UPPER EXTREMITY
19 Clavicle (collarbone)
20 Scapula
   (shoulder blade)
21 Humerus (arm)
22 Ulna ⎫
23 Radius ⎬ (forearm)
24 Carpal bones (wrist)
25 Metacarpals (palm)
26 Phalanges
   (finger bones)

THE MUSCULATURE

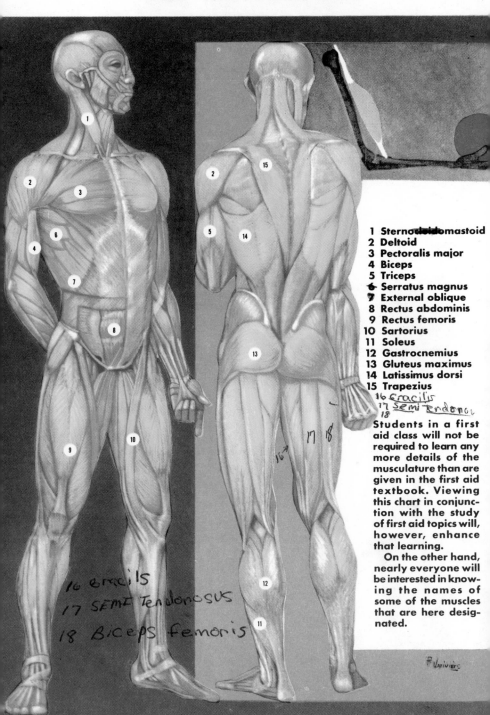

1 Sternocleidomastoid
2 Deltoid
3 Pectoralis major
4 Biceps
5 Triceps
6 Serratus magnus
7 External oblique
8 Rectus abdominis
9 Rectus femoris
10 Sartorius
11 Soleus
12 Gastrocnemius
13 Gluteus maximus
14 Latissimus dorsi
15 Trapezius
16 Gracilis
17 Semi-tendonor
18

Students in a first aid class will not be required to learn any more details of the musculature than are given in the first aid textbook. Viewing this chart in conjunction with the study of first aid topics will, however, enhance that learning.

On the other hand, nearly everyone will be interested in knowing the names of some of the muscles that are here designated.

16 Gracils
17 SEMI TenJonosus
18 Biceps femoris

THE INTERNAL ORGANS

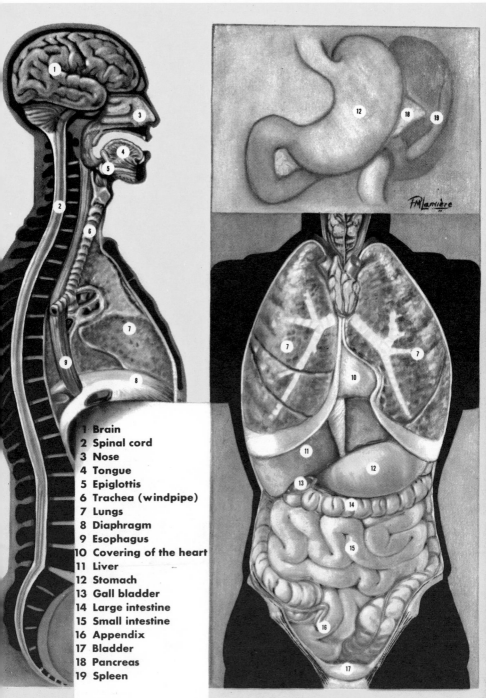

1 Brain
2 Spinal cord
3 Nose
4 Tongue
5 Epiglottis
6 Trachea (windpipe)
7 Lungs
8 Diaphragm
9 Esophagus
10 Covering of the heart
11 Liver
12 Stomach
13 Gall bladder
14 Large intestine
15 Small intestine
16 Appendix
17 Bladder
18 Pancreas
19 Spleen

Artist: P. M. Lariviere

POISONOUS SNAKES

Diamondback Rattlesnake

(Crotalus adamanteus)

found: From central coast region of North Carolina, along lower coastal plain through Florida, and westward to eastern Louisiana.

size: Up to 8 feet.

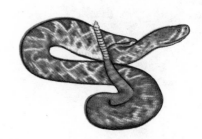

Timber Rattlesnake

(Crotalus horridus)

also called: Banded rattlesnake, mountain rattler, black rattler.

found: In uplands and mountains from southern Maine to northern Florida, and westward to central Texas.

size: Up to 6 feet. Average 4 feet.

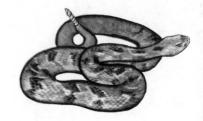

Massasauga

(Sistrurus catenatus)

also called: Pigmy rattlesnake.

found: Western New York and northwestern Pennsylvania westward to northeastern Kansas on the south, and southeastern Minnesota on the north. A sub-species extends into Texas, Arizona and Colorado.

size: Up to 3 feet.

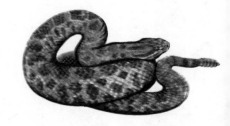

Artist: Doris M. Cochran, Ph.D.

POISONOUS SNAKES

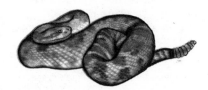

Pacific Rattlesnake
(Crotalus viridis oreganus)

found: British Columbia to southern California and Lower California; east to Idaho, Nevada, and Arizona.

size: Up to 5 feet.

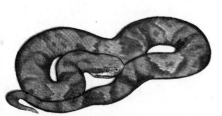

Water Moccasin
(Agkistrodon piscivorus)

also called: Cottonmouth and water pilot.

found: From southeastern Virginia, along coastal plains through Florida, and westward to central Texas; Mississippi Valley up to southern Illinois.

size: Up to 5 feet.

Copperhead
(Agkistrodon mokeson)

also called: Highland moccasin, rattlesnake pilot, coppersnake, and chunkhead.

found: Massachusetts to northern Florida, westward to Mississippi River in Illinois, and across to Texas. Found in hilly, rocky country and in lowlands; in walls, hedges, slab sawdust piles, haystacks, barns; even in villages and towns.

size: Up to 53 inches. Average 3 feet.

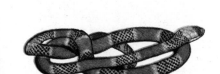

Coral Snake
(Micrurus fulvius)

also called: Harlequin and bead snake.

found: Along the coastal plains from central North Carolina, through Florida, westward to Texas, and up the Mississippi Valley to Indiana.

size: Up to 39 inches.

SOME POISONOUS PLANTS

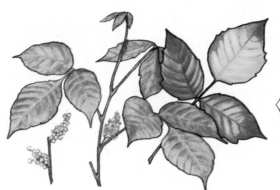

Common Poison Ivy
(Rhus radicans)

Grows as a small plant, a vine, and a shrub.

Grows everywhere in the United States except in California and parts of adjacent states. Eastern oak-leaf poison ivy is one of its varieties.

Leaves always consist of three glossy leaflets.

Also known as three-leaf ivy, poison creeper, climbing sumac, poison oak, markweed, picry, and mercury.

Western Poison Oak
(Rhus diversiloba)

Grows in shrub and, sometimes, vine form.

Grows in California and parts of adjacent states.

Sometimes called poison ivy, or yeara.

Leaves always consist of three leaflets.

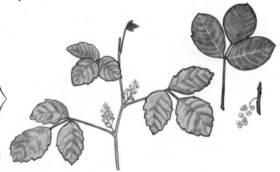

Poison Sumac
(Rhus vernix)

Grows as a woody shrub or small tree, five to twenty-five feet tall.

Grows in most of the eastern third of the United States.

Also known as swamp sumac, poison elder, poison ash, poison dogwood, and thunderwood.

NOTE: These plants belong to the same genus: *Rhus*. Since they contain the same poisonous substance, treatment for poisoning caused by them is the same for all.

Artist: Jane Roller

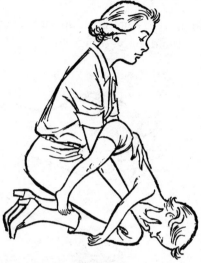

Fig. 52.2

3. Place the child on his back and use the middle
fingers of both hands to lift the lower jaw from
beneath and behind so that it "juts out." (Fig.
52.3)

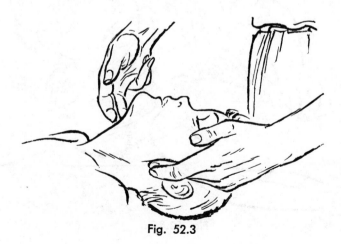

Fig. 52.3

4. Hold the jaw in the position described in Step 3, using one hand only. (Fig. 52.4)

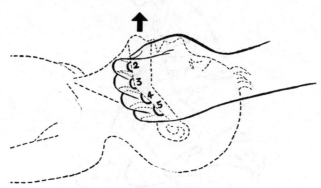

Fig. 52.4

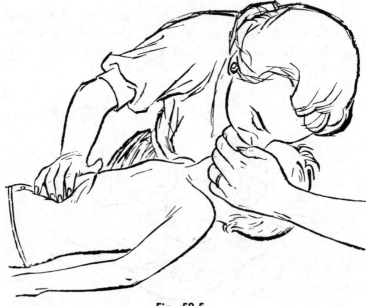

Fig. 52.5

5. Place your mouth over the child's mouth *and* nose, making a relatively leakproof seal, and breathe into the child with a smooth steady action until you observe the chest rise. As you start this action, move the free hand to the child's abdomen, between the navel and the ribs, and apply continuous moderate pressure to prevent the stomach from becoming filled with air. (Fig. 52.5)

6. When the lungs have been inflated, remove your lips from the child's mouth and nose and allow the lungs to empty. Repeat this cycle keeping one hand beneath the jaw and the other hand pressing on the stomach at all times. Continue at a rate of about 20 cycles per minute. After every 20 cycles the operator should rest long enough to take one deep breath. If at any time you feel resistance to your breathing into the child and the chest does not rise, repeat Step 2, then quickly resume mouth-to-mouth breathing.

The question often arises concerning a technique to use on adults when the chest is injured and compression of the chest would do further damage or when fractured upper extremities would eliminate the expansion phase of "push-pull" techniques. The mouth-to-mouth or mouth-to-nose technique may be used in these cases; however, the cycle should be slower than that used for children. Approximately 12 cycles per minute should be adequate. The lower jaw must be held in the "jutting out" position with both hands at all times.

3-Man Hammock Carry

Position of victim—supine

Step 1. All carriers kneel on the knee towards the victim's feet.

Step 2. No. 1 cradles the victim's head and shoulders with the top arm. The other arm is placed under the lower back.

Step 3. No. 2 slides his top arm under the victim's back *above* No. 1's bottom arm and his other arm just below the buttocks.

Step 4. No. 3 slides his top arm under the victim's thighs

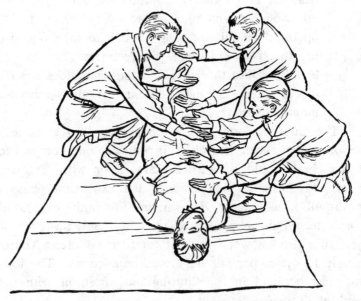

Fig. 53 Hammock carry step 1—position of bearers.

above No. 2's bottom arm. His other arm is placed under the victim's legs below the knees.

NOTE: The hands of carriers one and two should be placed about halfway under the body at this stage.

Step 5. At a signal, the victim is lifted to the carriers' knees and rested there while the hands are slid far enough under the victim to allow rotation of the hands *inward* to secure an interlocking grip.

Step 6. At the next signal, all carriers stand erect with the victim.

Step 7. To lower the victim to the ground, merely reverse the procedure.

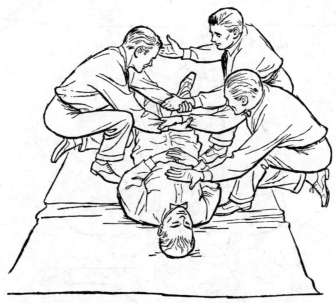

Fig. 54 Hammock carry—showing interlocking grip.

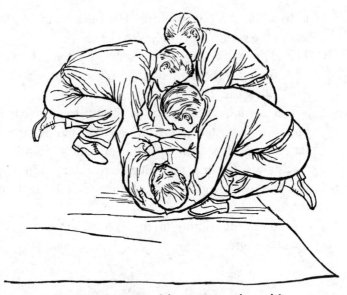

Fig. 55   Position of bearers—ready to lift.

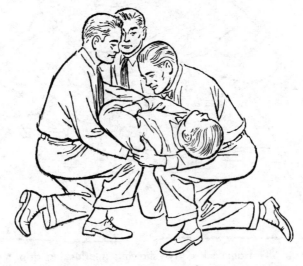

Fig. 56   Position of bearers—lifting victim to knees.

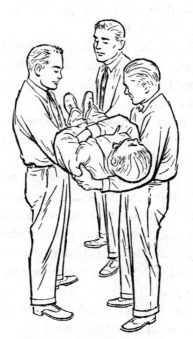

Fig. 57 Ready to carry.

Traction Blanket Lift (5 Men and Victim)

Position of victim—supine

Step 1. Pleat a standard army blanket in folds about 1-1½ ft. long and place on the floor just above the victim's head so that the pleated blanket will "feed out" from the bottom.

Step 2. Fold back the top pleat so that the man at the head and the two men at the shoulders can kneel on the fold.

Position of carriers:

Step 3. No. 1 takes the position on one or both knees and grasps the victim's head in the standard manner for applying traction.

Step 4. Nos. 2 and 3 kneel on one or both knees at the victim's shoulders, placing one hand flat under the shoulder blade and the other in the armpit.

Step 5. Nos. 4 and 5 grasp the bottom pleat of the blanket and pull the blanket under the victim while Nos. 1, 2, and 3 hold the upper portion of the victim's body in place.

Step 6. Roll the blanket tightly at the sides until it fits the contour of the victim's body.

Step 7. Nos. 2 and 3 (on opposite sides) grasp the blanket with the top hands at the shoulder and the bottom hands at lower back. Nos. 4 and 5 grasp blanket with top hands at the hips and lower hands at the legs (below knees). No. 1 remains at the head, holding slight traction.

Step 8. At a signal, Nos. 2, 3, 4, and 5 *lean* back in opposite directions using the back muscles and body weight. This will lift the victim 6 to 8 inches from the floor so that a litter can be slid underneath. Same procedure with victim in *prone* position.

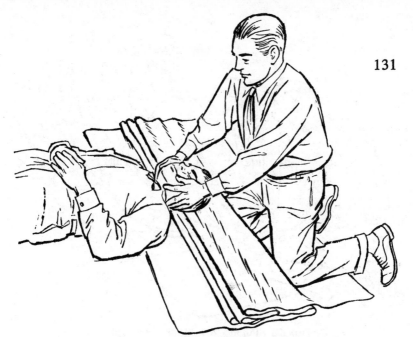

Fig. 58   Step 1—placing blanket under victim.

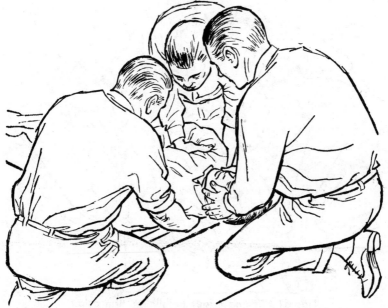

Fig. 59   Step 2—holding victim against the pull of the blanket.

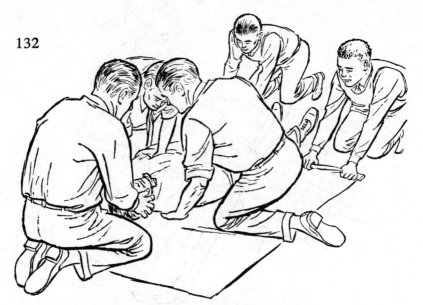

Fig. 60 Pulling the blanket through.

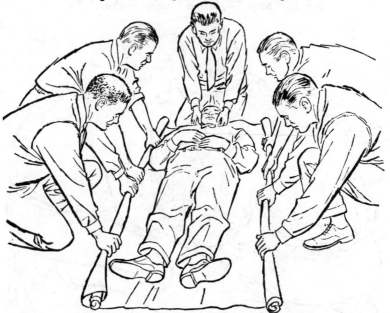

Fig. 61 Rolling edges tightly for firm grip.

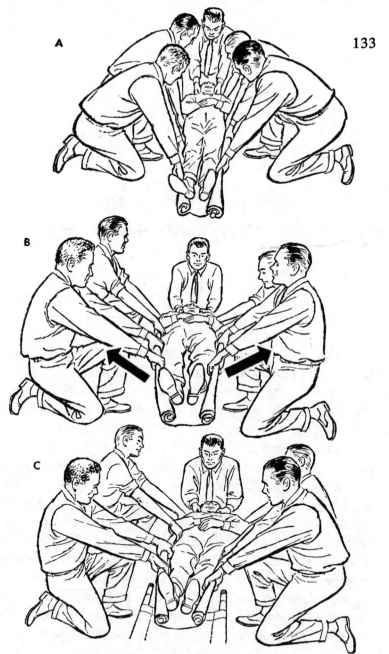

Fig. 62   A. Blanket fits contour of body.   B. Bearers lean backward.
C. Lowering victim to litter.

ADVANCED FIRST AID
THEORY AND SKILLS

CHAPTER XI

THE HUMAN BODY

The body framework is divided into the head, neck, trunk, and limbs, or extremities.

There are more than 200 bones in the body. These give shape to the body, protect vital organs, and contribute toward effective motion.

At any place where the edges of two bones are in close contact, there is a joint. At many joints, such as those of the shoulder and fingers, the motions of rotating or bending are possible. Here tough connective tissue bands called ligaments extend from one bone end to the end of the adjacent bone, enclosing the joint and holding the bone ends in place. If great force is applied at a joint, the ligaments may be overstretched or torn; and perhaps the surrounding muscles, blood vessels, and nerves suffer injury too.

Motion is not always associated with a joint. For example, the skull has 14 bones in the facial part and 8 bones in the rest of the head (excluding the tiny bones of the middle ear) but only one bone—the lower jaw —is movable. The other bones are either fused together in adulthood or are tightly joined by connective tissue. Further, they do not have muscle attachments acting upon them to cause motion. Likewise in the chest and pelvis are certain joints that permit little or no motion.

The body substance, or tissue, consists of different kinds of living cells, such as muscle, nerve, and gland cells, and other material. For example, blood tissue consists in part of living cells, such as white blood cells, and of other substance, such as the fluid part. Bone tissue is composed of living cells interspersed in hard material formed by the cells. Skin tissue is composed of deep-lying living cells and overlying dead cells.

The Skeletal System

The skull

The skull consists of the upper and back part (the cranium, which encloses the brain) and the facial bones. These bones heal readily in case of fracture, but sometimes it is necessary to reposition the fractured parts.

The backbone

The backbone (spinal column) is composed of 33 bones called vertebrae. There are 7 neck, 12 chest, and 5 lumbar vertebrae. The lowest-lying 9 vertebrae form the sacrum and coccyx or tail bone. The sacrum consists of 5 fused vertebrae and forms a part of the pelvis. The remaining 4 vertebrae form the coccyx. The upper 24 are separated by plates or discs of cartilage or gristle, and a slight degree of bending is possible at each joint. Occasionally because of a blow, twisting, or heavy lifting, a disc may slip out of place. The backbone encases the spinal cord. If a vertebra or disc is fractured or dislocated, the spinal cord may be injured so that sometimes paralysis or loss of sensation results in body parts below. Occasionally, because of a fall or violent forward bending of the trunk, a vertebra is compressed in such a fashion as to bring the upper and lower surfaces of the vertebra closer together. This is called a compression fracture.

The breastbone

The breastbone (sternum) is a flat bone. At its upper end the collarbones are attached. The 24 ribs are fastened to the chest vertebrae in back and, with the exception of the lowest two on each side, to the breastbone in front. The shoulder blades lie in the back wall of the chest. Each one has a socket for the arm bone, and also an attachment to the outer end of the collarbone.

The pelvis

The pelvis consists of a girdle of fused bones. It supports the backbone and has a socket for each thigh bone. Fractures of the pelvis most commonly are located in the front portion, and cause discomfort in the lower abdomen or crotch upon walking.

The upper extremities

There is one bone in the arm, two in the forearm, eight

in the wrist, five in the palm, two in the thumb, and three in each of the other digits of the hand.

The lower extremities

There is one bone in the thigh and two in the leg. The ankle joint consists of the lower ends of the two leg bones and a foot bone, the talus. In the back portion of the foot, there are 7 bones including the talus; 5 bones that form the long part of the foot; 2 in the great toe; and 3 in each of the other toes. The kneecap, a bone somewhat larger than a silver dollar, lies in front of the knee joint.

The thigh bone and the shin bone have plates of gristle (cartilage) over their ends at the knee joints. The cartilage may be broken in case of a strong, twisting force at the knee joint. Fractures of the thigh bone may occur at any point. The commonest point is at the upper end, through the neck of the thigh bone.

The Circulatory System

The circulatory system includes the blood circulation system and the lymph system. The blood circulation system includes the heart, the blood vessels, and the blood. There are three kinds of blood vessels: arteries, capillaries, and veins. Arteries carry blood *from* the heart toward the capillaries. They have relatively thick walls and branch into progressively smaller arteries until they merge into the capillaries. Capillaries are microscopic, thin-walled vessels. The exchange of food, oxygen, and wastes between the body cells and the blood occurs through the capillary walls. The veins are those vessels which carry blood from the capillaries *toward* the heart.

The heart

The heart is largely muscle tissue. It has a receiving chamber and a pumping chamber on both the left and right sides. Valves regulate the flow of blood. The left chamber receives blood rich in oxygen from the lungs. The left pumping chamber sends this blood into the great artery, the aorta, from which it goes to all parts of the body. After distribution throughout the body, the blood returns to the right receiving chamber, then to the right pumping chamber. From here it is pumped into the lungs, thereby starting the process over again.

The heart beats about 70-75 times per minute in most adults when they are at rest. Generally, the rate is lower in the morning, when body temperature is usually between 97 and 98 degrees, than in the late afternoon when the temperature is above 98 degrees. Generally, the heart rate increases when body temperature rises, as with fever. Along the arteries, heart contractions cause a pulsation, which may be *counted readily at the wrist*.

The blood

The blood consists of a fluid part (plasma) and of suspended solid microscopic particles (red cells, white cells, and platelets). Red cells transport oxygen, white cells combat germs, and platelets assist in the process of blood clotting. The plasma contains dissolved chemicals, such as nutriment, carbon dioxide, hormones, gamma globulin, other proteins, and waste products. Most of the antibodies of the blood, useful in defense against germs and their harmful products, are contained in the gamma globulin fraction of the plasma.

The Lymph System

This consists of a network of small vessels with no pumping action. The fluid flows along slowly because of gravity, to some extent, and because of muscular contractions in surrounding muscle. When blood passes through the capillaries, it is under pressure and some of the blood *fluid* escapes through the thin capillary walls into the surrounding tissue. The solid particles cannot escape, except that the white cells sometimes wriggle through when attracted by germs. Part of the escaped fluid returns into the capillaries; but part of it flows slowly along, forming a film around the tissue cells. It drains into the lymph vessels, which merge into larger vessels and finally empty into certain veins. The lymph vessels are enlarged at certain places called lymph nodes; here many white cells are present and act against germs that are in the fluid. Infection may sometimes be indicated by a red streak along the forearm or leg, for example, or by tender lumps in the armpit or groin. These symptoms indicate an inflammation along the lymph channel and in the lymph nodes. Sometimes the conditioning is wrongly called "blood poisoning."

The Respiratory System

The respiratory passages consist of the nose, throat, windpipe (trachea), bronchial tubes, and lungs. Surrounding the lungs is a double layer of thin tissue called the pleura. In the lungs the branches of the bronchial tubes terminate in microscopic air sacs. These thin-walled sacs are surrounded by capillaries, which pass oxygen to the blood and receive carbon dioxide from the blood.

The oxygen joins chemically with the hemoglobin contained in the red cells. When red cells reach the body cells, oxygen leaves the blood and unites in the surrounding tissue with food elements, such as carbohydrate products. This union is essentially a process of slow burning that liberates energy as heat or muscle energy; carbon dioxide is one of the by-products.

In the breathing process, chest capacity is increased in two ways. First, the muscles in the chest wall contract, thereby expanding the chest. Meanwhile, the diaphragm muscles contract, causing the diaphragm to *descend*. Since air at sea level exerts almost 15 pounds of pressure per square inch, it rushes into the lungs when the chest capacity increases. At each breath, the average adult takes in about a pint of air. The average adult male has about 3 quarts or less of air in his lungs unless he takes a deep breath, when he would add about two quarts more. Air contains about 21 percent oxygen when it enters the lungs and about 16 percent when it leaves. It is likely that if only about one-half pint were breathed each time, the amount would be sufficient during rest.

The Nervous System

The nervous system consists of the brain, spinal cord, and innumerable nerves that supply the various body parts. Nerves that carry impulses effecting the action of muscles or glands are called *motor* nerves. Nerves that carry impulses from body parts because of a change in conditions of the part or because of an unusual condition are called *sensory* nerves. For example, when a bone is broken, sensory

nerves carry impulses from nerve endings in the damaged region to the spinal cord. From there, motor nerves transmit the impulse to the muscles surrounding the bone, and cause muscle spasm. In this example, the sensory impulse never reaches the conscious centers of the brain and the body reaction is a reflex before the person is aware of pain. Sensory nerve impulses constantly pass along from a body organ to the spinal cord, and then travel along motor nerves to cause changes in the activity of internal organs and blood vessels.

Sometimes sensory nerves do carry along impulses that finally reach the conscious centers in the brain with resulting sensations of pain, cold, pressure, and the like.

In addition to sensory and motor nerves, there are many *association* nerves, which connect one nerve with another and relay impulses along. The brain is well supplied with association nerves.

If a nerve is cut, the part beyond degenerates. However, in some cases—not always—the nerve will grow along the path of the degenerated part. Eventually, sensation and movement may return to normal.

Muscles and Tendons

Muscle cells have the ability to shorten or contract. The muscle cells that cause motion at joints have a framework of soft connective tissue and thus form a muscle band. The biceps muscle of the arm is such a muscle band made up of numerous muscle cells and connective tissue. Muscles that cause joint motion are attached to bones above and below the joint. Near their points of attachment, the bands consist largely of tough connective tissue with few or no muscle cells; these portions of the muscle bands are called *tendons*. Suppose that one end of a band is attached to the shoulder blade and the other end is attached to a forearm bone, on the palm side. When the muscle contracts slightly, the elbow bends considerably.

Many muscles are under control of the will; others are not. For example, the blood vessels, especially the smaller arteries, contain muscle cells or fibrils (FI brils) that encircle the inside of the vessel wall. When the cells contract, the vessel constricts so that less blood can go through.

Many muscles seldom relax completely; they regularly are in a state of slight contraction. Sometimes the degree of habitual contraction is affected by the emotions; a person's mental tension may affect the tension of the muscles in a complicated way through nerve impulses, probably largely or completely unknown to the person.

The Digestive System

The digestive tube consists of the mouth, throat, esophagus, stomach, small intestine, and large intestine. The large intestine is the colon; its lower portion is the rectum. The entire tube in adults is almost 30 feet long, the small intestine being about 22 feet and the large intestine about 5 feet. In addition to the food tube, the digestive system includes many other organs that aid in digestion in some way—the salivary glands, the tongue, pancreas, and liver. The pancreas and liver also have additional functions beyond those related to digestion. Digestion is the breakdown of food into simpler chemicals that are soluble and will pass through the walls of the food tube into the capillaries. This breakdown occurs largely in the small intestine. An enormous number of germs are present in the food tube—the mouth and intestines especially. If the intestines are cut, germs escape and cause inflammation of the lining of the abdomen. This lining is called peritoneum, and the inflammation is peritonitis.

The large bowel eliminates unabsorbed food and certain excretions from the liver. There are a number of organs that take material from the blood and discharge it directly or indirectly from the body. These include the kidneys (urine), the lungs (carbon dioxide), the skin (perspiration), and the liver (bile). Some parts of the bile are used by the body; others are waste products.

The *endocrine glands* discharge *hormones* into the blood, affecting body processes. Among the endocrine glands are the pituitary, thyroid and parathyroid, the pancreas, the adrenal, and the male and female gonads. Many of these glands form several kinds of hormones.

CHAPTER XII

SPECIAL WOUNDS

Wounds with foreign bodies should be regarded as being dangerously contaminated. Dirt, pieces of glass, metal shavings, and bits of cloth and wood often are present in wounds. Unless the wounds are cleaned thoroughly, infection is virtually certain. Not infrequently, foreign material harbors tetanus germs. For example, a study of street dust in Baltimore, Maryland, showed that about 15 percent of the samples contained this germ.

Sometimes a thorn or tiny splinter of wood penetrates the skin. If you elect to remove it, first wash the hands thoroughly and apply an antiseptic to the skin. Then, sterilize a knife point or needle by flaming it before attempting the removal.

If a sizable foreign body is firmly wedged in a wound and protrudes from the surface, it is usually best to leave it there, pending medical attention. Removal may not only cause pain and profuse bleeding but will give the physician less basis for determining underlying damage.

Fishhooks sometimes penetrate the skin, especially that of the hand. If the barb extends under the skin, the wisest course is to have the physician remove it.

Wounds Extending Deep into the Body

When wounds extend deep into the head, neck, chest, or abdomen, the paramount objective of first aid is to see that the victim does not suffer additional harm before he receives medical care. Wounds must be protected from contamination, bleeding stopped, breathing difficulty controlled as far as possible, and immobility of affected parts maintained. It is often best, by far, to summon a physician to the scene rather than move the patient.

If the accident occurs far from medical facilities, the first aider should foresee possible difficulties, such as the effect of swelling upon breathing if the nose and mouth passages are severely mutilated, or of injury to the lower abdomen upon urination. In such cases, prudent haste in bringing the victim to medical care is indicated.

Since the victim probably will have surgery, food should not be given. Fluid likewise should be withheld. With shock as a danger, the foot of the bed or other support should be raised 8 to 12 inches. If breathing difficulty develops, raise the head and shoulders on pillows.

Sometimes air passes through a chest wound with each inspiration and expiration. Such air exchange in any direction should be stopped completely by placing sufficient dressing material firmly against the wound. The victim should lie on the wounded side.

For an abdominal wound, give no food or water, and consider possible urinary difficulty. Rarely do the intestines protrude from the wound. However, if they do protrude, they will become gangrenous unless kept moist. Sterile cloths, wet with boiled water, should be placed over the wound. The water should be at body temperature, tested by pouring some on the forearm. In the absence of sterile supplies, the closest possible approach to sterile conditions should be sought. No attempt should be made to push the intestines back into the abdomen. If these victims are transported, they may retch and vomit, thus forcing out more intestine. Fortunately, the problem is extremely rare.

Gunshot Wounds

The surface injury from gunshot may vary from the almost undetectable to the extremely extensive. Penetration may be deep or only slight. First aid methods are not different from those already considered, but several points deserve mention. Police must be notified.

The surface wound may be small. In such case, if the victim has few complaints, the first aider may think that the injury is slight even though a highpowered weapon was used. Delayed evidence of serious internal injury, such as slow bleeding, will appear.

Always consider the possibility that the missile caused a fracture. Sometimes a shotgun, loaded with slugs, causes an extensive wound that diverts thought from the possibility of fracture. If an extremity has been injured, splint it before attempting transportation. This procedure is definitely helpful, even if only the soft tissue is damaged.

The use of blank cartridges is not without danger. If a gun loaded with them is discharged at someone close by, he may suffer serious injury. Deaths have resulted from the mis-use of blank cartridges.

Animal Bites and Stings

Because animal bites carry germs from the animal's mouth and the victim's skin and clothing into the wound, infection with any of a variety of germs is possible. The wounds are lacerations or punctures; and in some cases, tetanus and rabies are added dangers. The bite of a human sometimes causes a persistent infection unless properly treated.

Bites with danger of rabies

Warm-blooded animals are susceptible to rabies. The disease is spread to man most often by dogs and occasionally by cats.

The bite of a rabid animal *may* not cause rabies in the victim; but if symptoms *do* appear in man, the disease is invariably fatal. The danger of rabies is greater when the wounds involve the head or neck, but the illness can also occur if the sick animal licks any opening in the skin. Rabid dogs may be unusually active, irritable, or clearly dangerous, or they may be quiet, stuporous, or affectionate.

In case of animal bite, rabies can be prevented by immunization of the victim. The procedure currently used requires 14 or more injections. Because some bites do not transmit rabies, it is best to determine whether the animal has the disease before commencing the injections. If infectious, the dog will die within two weeks; then the brain tissue can be examined to find distinctive evidence of rabies. Immunization may be postponed during this period unless the danger seems especially great—as with severe and lacerating wounds or with wounds of the face and neck.

The animal should be confined in the facilities of a veterinarian or the animal rescue society. Here it presents no risk. If the animal is killed at once after the bite, there is no chance to observe whether it is ill. Further, if the head is examined, the distinctive evidences are less often present in the brain tissue than after the disease has run its course. Sometimes, in order to protect others, a dog must be killed at once. If this is necessary, avoid shooting it in the head.

A new method for vaccinating healthy dogs against rabies is available. One injection apparently leads to protection for four years or more and will also prevent the dog from transmitting rabies.

First aid. In case of animal bite, wash the wound thoroughly to remove the saliva. Use a gauze compress and a solution of soap and water to scrub the wound; then rinse it with clean running water and apply a sterile dressing.

Always consult a physician at once. The first aid cleansing does not insure against the development of rabies or tetanus, but it is of some help. The physician will then decide whether it is safe to postpone immunization of the victim while the dog is under study and whether preventive measures against tetanus are necessary. He will also treat the wounds more effectively.

Snake bites

There are four kinds of poisonous snakes in the United States. Pit vipers are rattlesnakes, copperheads, and cottonmouth moccasins. The other poisonous snake is the coral snake. The pit vipers have a pit on each side of the head between the eyes and the nostrils. The coral snake, found along the coast and lowlands of the Southeast, is small; it chews rather than bites and cannot readily attach to large surfaces, such as the forearm and calf. Its potent venom affects the nervous system, whereas that of the pit vipers affects the blood circulatory system. The fatality rate from *untreated* poisonous snake bites probably is between 10 and 15 percent. Most snake bite fatalities in this country are caused by rattlesnakes; they inject much venom if they are large and if they have not discharged their supply recently.

Prevention. In snake-infested country, watch where you step, where you place your hands, and where you sit. Wear high boots or stout leggings, because over half of all bites are below midcalf. Take care when picking berries and flowers, and when climbing ledges, where your hands may reach up and disturb a resting snake.

Symptoms. Pain is immediate if pit viper venom is injected. The poisoned part soon swells and discoloration appears. Coral snake venom causes only slight burning pain and mild swelling at the wound. The bite of a nonvenomous snake gives little pain and produces no swelling beyond the usual for any wound, nor any general reaction except perhaps an emotional one. Pit vipers inflict one or two puncture wounds. They may introduce tetanus germs as well as venom.

With absorption of the poison, there is general weakness, shortness of breath, nausea and vomiting, a weak and rapid pulse, and sometimes dimness of vision. Unconsciousness may occur. If the poison was injected directly into the blood stream, these signs appear quickly. Otherwise absorption is slower and reactions may become marked only after an hour or two.

First aid. If the snake is nonpoisonous, first aid is the same as for ordinary wounds. These bites are scratch-like rather than punctures. Watch the victim for a time, because the emotional reaction may cause him to faint.

If the snake is *poisonous*:

1. Have the victim stop muscular activity at once.

2. Tie a constricting band firmly above the bite if it is on an extremity. This band should be tight enough to prevent the return flow of blood in the surface vessels, but not enough to shut off the deep-lying vessels. If properly adjusted, there will be some oozing from the wound.

3. Sterilize a knife blade with a match flame and make incisions. Try with one of them to get into the venom deposit point, remembering that the snake strikes downward and the fangs retract. Crosscuts, about one-fourth inch long, may be made at each fang mark and over the suspected deposit point. Make shallow cuts through the skin in the crossways direction; longitudinal cuts may be deeper. Muscles and nerves run in a longitudinal direction and a deep crosscut may sever them. Beware of cutting muscles and nerves of the fingers, hands, or wrist, for they lie immediately below the skin, and their injury may cause much disability.

4. Apply suction, using the mouth or suction cup.

The venom is not a stomach poison, but it is advisable to rinse the fluid from the mouth. Some poison might be absorbed along an infected gum margin, but the effects would be mild and local. Continue suction for an hour or more.

5. Get medical care. If transportation is necessary, keep the victim lying down, with the injured part somewhat lower than the rest of the body. During relief-from-suction periods, apply ice or cold water, if possible, to the part involved. This gives some relief from pain and may slow the absorption of poison into the system.

Scorpion stings

Scorpions, spiders, chiggers, and ticks all are members of the same animal class (arachnids). Scorpions have 8 legs, a pair of appendages at the head end that somewhat resemble those of a crab, an elongated body, and a slender, segmented tail, which may curl up. The stinger is located at the tip of the tail. Adults of some species are more than 3 inches long. Scorpions are most common in the southwestern part of the U. S. They are found in cool and damp houses, debris, and under loose banks rather than in the hot sun.

Most species of scorpions in this country do not inject a human toxin; therefore the large share of stings are not dangerous. The usual sting results in some local swelling and discoloration, perhaps pain like that of a wasp sting for a half an hour or more, and sometimes allergic reaction.

The sting of the more dangerous species of scorpions causes little or no swelling and discoloration, but locally there may be a tingling or burning sensation. In the adult, considerable discomfort ensues. Death, although unlikely, occurs occasionally in infants and young children, and might conceivably occur in older, infirm people. The poison acts mainly on the nervous system. A badly poisoned small child becomes restless; soon nausea, then cramp of the abdominal and other muscles, and perhaps convulsions develop.

First aid.

1. If the sting is on a finger or toe, immediately apply at the base, a tight, narrow constricting band. If the sting is higher, use a wider band above the sting on the heart side. Remove the band after it has been in place for five minutes.

2. Pack the area generously in ice for two hours. Keep the affected extremity somewhat lower than the rest of the body during this two-hour period.

3. Provide sufficient body covering to maintain comfort.
   If the sting does not involve one of the four extremities, ice applications are the only local first aid measure.

4. Obtain medical attention. Helpful measures against pain and systemic symptoms are available. The sting wound may need treatment to prevent infection.

Cuts and suction are of little value because of the minute quantity of toxin injected.

Black widow spider bites

Black widow spiders are common in the southern half of the country, but are found occasionally in the northern half. The adult female's body is about a half-inch long, shiny black, usually with red hourglass marking on the underside of the abdomen. Infrequently, there are other markings or no red whatever. The males are about one-fourth the size of the females and have several white stripes as well as the hourglass on the abdomen and a red stripe on the middle of the back. The young often have a row of red dots along the back. These spiders are found outdoors under stones, in hollow stumps, woodpiles, and other protected places; indoors they are found in a wide variety of places where there is some dampness.

The brown widow spider also has an hourglass marking on the abdomen, but it is dull orange against a brown body; this species is harmless, but in rare cases there is an allergic reaction to the material injected.

Symptoms. The bite of a black widow causes redness and only slight swelling locally. Pain commences at once and is exceedingly severe, spreading throughout the body. Profuse perspiration, nausea, and difficulties in breathing and speaking may develop. Painful cramps of abdominal and other muscles are common. Almost all cases recover, but the course of illness for a day or more may be stormy.

First aid. The first aid is the same as that for scorpion stings. If after several hours the victim has not had medical attention, hot wet applications or a hot bath may give some relief if muscle pains are severe.

Tarantula bites

Tarantulas are hairy spiders. Adult females may measure up to about three inches in length, not including the legs; those in this country are somewhat smaller. They are found in the southwestern section of the U. S. These tarantulas are quite harmless, but occasionally a victim will have an allergic reaction to the injected material. The bite usually feels like a pinprick. Some tarantulas that come into the country with imported fruit or otherwise may be more poisonous, causing rather marked pain and local redness and swelling. Deaths are extremely rare.

First aid. First aid for bites from non-poisonous tarantulas is the same as for any insect bite: cleansing followed by a dressing. For the bite of a tarantula, the same measures as recommended for scorpion sting are used.

Irritation from chiggers

Chiggers are the larval stage of a mite, having hatched from tiny brown eggs laid in moist soil. The irritation produced by chiggers results from a fluid they inject; it does not appear until an hour or more after exposure and commonly persists several days. Chiggers *do not* burrow under the skin.

Prevention. Chiggers are most common in the South, especially in regions of lush vegetation and moisture. Wearing high shoes or boots is of some protective value. A time-honored chigger repellent, not entirely satisfactory, has been the sprinkling of sulfur upon the clothes before expected exposure. Other measures are, rinsing clothes in 5 percent dimethyl phthalate in 2 percent soapy water and a 5 percent benzyl benzoate solution in water.

Chiggers usually do not attach themselves for an hour or more after they reach the body. Therefore, bathing promptly after exposure, using a brush and soapy water, may eliminate them. If undiluted denatured alcohol or sulfur ointment is applied to the skin after bathing, the protection is increased.

First aid. Once the bite is inflicted, measures are only palliative. Application of ice water gives some relief. Bathing the affected parts with baking soda solution, ammonia water, or strong alcohol solution also has some value.

Insect bites and stings

Today many commercial insect repellents are available. First aid measures are not entirely effective because the bite wounds extend beneath the skin. A paste made of baking soda and cold cream or a compress moistened with ammonia water gives some relief; calamine lotion also relieves the itching. For bee and wasp stings, the immediate application of ice or ice water gives relief and probably slows the absorption from the site. These applications also have value for any insect bite. For people known to be allergic to bee or wasp poison and for those who have other allergies to specific insects, the use of a tight constricting band is advised in case the sting is on an extremity; and in any case, ice should be applied, pending medical care.

Tick bites

Ticks are flat, usually brown, and about one-fourth inch long; they have 8 legs. In some cases they can transmit germs of several diseases, including Rocky Mountain

Spotted Fever, a disease occurring in the East as well as the West. They adhere tenaciously to the skin or scalp. There is some evidence that the longer an infected one remains attached, the greater is the chance that it will transmit the disease.

First aid. Although use of tweezers for removal of a tick, or application of heat to its body, as by a lighted cigarette, have been attempted often, these methods may leave tick parts in the wound or may injure the skin. A better method is to cover the tick with heavy oil (mineral, salad, or machine) to close its breathing pores. It may disengage at once; if not, allow the oil to remain in place for a half an hour. Then remove the tick carefully with tweezers, taking time so that all parts come away. Gently scrub the area thoroughly with soap and water because the disease germs may be present on the skin.

Marine life that causes skin irritation

Along the seacoasts many cases of severe skin irritation and poisoning are caused by marine animals, such as the Portuguese man-of-war. These animals inject irritating substances. They may cause enough pain to weaken the person greatly; occasionally severe shock develops.

First aid. If an animal part, such as a bit of the tentacles of jellyfish or the man-of-war, remains embedded in the skin, remove it at once by washing with water containing enough sand to form a soupy mixture. Otherwise, wash with cold salt-water, and then place the involved extremity in hot water for 30 to 60 minutes. The application of half-strength household ammonia solution followed by a paste of bicarbonate of soda and cold cream may be tried, but probably immersion in hot water gives as much relief.

CHAPTER XIII

COMMON EMERGENCIES—PART TWO

Appendicitis

This disease may occur at any age. Pain is almost always present in the right lower part of the abdomen, or the upper part especially at first, or is distributed throughout. Nausea and vomiting may be present. Fever seldom is high at first. Mild or marked constipation is common; occasionally bowel movements are normal or there may be mild diarrhea. Other diseases may give similar evidence; but with abdominal pain, quick action is necessary. The constipation sometimes is regarded erroneously as the cause of the discomfort and a laxative is administered. The effect is to defer obtaining medical attention and to increase the chance of rupture of the appendix.

First aid

Obtain medical attention immediately. Meanwhile, do not give a laxative, and withhold food and water. An ice bag placed over the appendix region may relieve discomfort; but it probably does not affect the course of the disease and should not mislead one into thinking that the disease is abating. Do not apply heat to the abdomen.

Blisters

Blood blisters and water blisters may be caused by pinching and chafing. They involve the palm, fingers, ankle, and feet regions most often.

First aid

Small collections of water or blood will be absorbed gradually by the body if the inciting pressure is relieved. Should the blister be raised and you decide to open it, first wash the part thoroughly with soap and water; then as additional precaution, apply an antiseptic to the skin. Sterilize a needle in an open flame and puncture the blister at its edge. Using a sterile gauze pad, apply pressure along the margin of the blister to remove the fluid; then place a sterile dressing over the area. If the blister already has burst, wash the part gently with soap and water and apply a sterile dressing. Self-care should not be attempted when the blister fluid lies deep in the palm.

Boils and Styes

Styes involve the margins of the eyelids, and boils are commonest on the back of the neck, about the nostrils, and on the extremities. They are caused by germs that enter from the skin surface, and are rubbed in by clothing, the hands, or other pressures.

People exposed to dust, dirt, oils, asphalt, and irritating chemicals are likely to develop boils unless they cleanse the skin frequently. Sometimes germs are rubbed down into several hair follicles, thus causing multiple boils, or an original boil may break, distributing many germs that penetrate the skin at several points.

People who are diabetic, aged, infirm, or infected with circulatory disease should especially beware of boils. The appearance of boils may be a clue that diabetes is present. Styes are said to be more common in people who need glasses or a change of lens, because they rub the eyes more often.

First aid

1. Do not squeeze a boil. Pressure upon it may drive germs into the circulatory system and can cause internal abscesses or a bone infection.

2. Keep the affected part as quiet and free from pressure as possible to promote healing and lessen the chance that the germs will work into the circulatory system. Take particular care against pressing or picking at boils of the nostrils, upper lip, and about the eyes, because here the circulation drains into the brain region.

3. Discomfort from small boils may be relieved with wet compresses. Apply Epsom salt solution, one tablespoonful to a pint of warm water, at 15-minute intervals. Packs should not be applied to facial boils except under medical direction.

4. If a boil breaks, wipe the pus away with a sterile pad wet with rubbing alcohol. Work from the normal skin toward the boil and pus; then apply a sterile dressing.

Convulsions In Young Children

Convulsions occur with many diseases. If the child has previously been healthy and is on a good diet, the most likely cause is an infection. Convulsions may appear at any time during the acute stage, or be the first evidence of such illnesses as tonsillitis, whooping cough, scarlet fever, and pneumonia. Among other causes are low blood calcium (as in rickets), poisons (especially lead), congenital defects, concussion, and lack of oxygen because of some interference with air flow. Convulsions are seldom, if ever, caused by teething, by worms (in this country, at least), or by over-eating in itself. Some children mimic convulsions excellently to gain their objectives.

Symptoms

The convulsion manifests itself as muscle spasms and twitching. All degrees of severity are seen. Sometimes only a twitching of the eyeballs is noticed; in other cases, the spasms involve the entire body. The attack may last from a few seconds to many minutes, and may recur repeatedly. The child is left in a stuporous condition or falls asleep.

First aid

1. Provide bed rest and quiet. Do not cover the child excessively, because he may have a fever. Do not exhibit alarm to the child.
2. Call a doctor. Meanwhile do not give an enema, bath, or warm packs unless specifically advised to do so. These measures are less often used now than

formerly and should be undertaken only when so directed.

3. If it is clear that a convulsion is being mimicked, be casually indifferent and matter-of-fact; show no alarm. The parents should discuss the incident with the family physician.

Hernia (Rupture)

In the front wall of the abdomen, part-way up the groin from the crotch, muscular effort, lifting, and other activities sometimes cause a loop of bowel to push from the abdominal cavity and cause a protrusion or bulge to appear at the weak spot. This condition is a hernia, or rupture. Other places where a hernia may appear are in the scar of an abdominal operation, at the navel, and just below the groin at the crotch. Hernia may affect the strong and the weak, the young and the old. It is more common to the obese but is by no means confined to them. During the first weeks, the rupture may cause some pain; later there might be less discomfort. The bulge generally disappears when the patient lies down, and reappears when he rises. As time goes on, the area increases, or works along certain paths, and the rupture almost always becomes worse. There is also the danger that constriction effects may shut off the blood supply of the loop of bowel, necessitating an emergency operation, since the bowel part will not survive long without blood.

First aid

1. When a rupture is noted, refrain from further lifting and vigorous activity, and seek medical at-

tention. Do not press on the bulge to force it back, because the path is seldom straight, and the pressure may damage the bowel. The protrusion probably will subside if the victim lies down.

2. If the bulge does not subside when the victim lies down, cold applications with cloths saturated with water may be effective. If these fail, the knee-chest maneuver may be tried. Lie on the abdomen, and bring the knees up under the chest so that the buttocks are high. Should these efforts fail, lie on the back until medical care is available.

Plant Poisoning

The commonest offenders are poison ivy, poison oak, and poison sumac. Among hundreds of others that cause occasional cases of poisoning are the primrose, smartweed, nettle, and cowhage; instances of poisoning have been reported from the tomato, potato, ragweed, geranium, and chrysanthemum plants. However, for the average person, the ones to study and avoid, are the first-named above. Virtually everyone can become sensitized to the poison they contain.

The active substance in the poison-ivy group is an oleoresin called urushiol. This substance is contained in the sap, leaves, fruit, flowers, roots, and bark, but apparently not in the pollen or wood. It does not evaporate except in temperatures far above those tolerable to man; therefore, one cannot be poisoned merely by close proximity except possibly when soot from a burning plant falls upon the skin.

While some people are not sensitive to the substance

upon first contact, this contact may cause sensitivity to later exposure. The sensitivity of any person varies at different times, and probably diminishes if there are no later exposures. A person may withstand exposure at one time and develop severe poisoning upon exposure the next time.

The degree of exposure is an important factor. Although some people develop poisoning from the slightest contact, in general the danger increases when exposure is vigorous to broken and abraded leaves and other parts that release the chemical upon the skin. The hazard is greatest in the spring and summer when the sap is most abundant.

Eating leaves or fruit in order to gain immunity, as is sometimes done, is exceedingly unwise. The administration of poison-ivy extracts to desensitize the person has not been altogether satisfactory. Such desensitization procedures must be started many months before the expected exposures, and probably are most effective and least likely to cause reactions when taken on a year-round basis.

Identifying the plants

The common poison ivy is found throughout the country except possibly in Nevada and California; it is also called the eastern poison ivy. The oakleaf ivy occurs in the southeastern states, and the western poison oak in the three Coastal states. All of these plants may occur as vines or as shrubs. The common ivy is usually a vine, the other two are usually shrubs, growing three to five feet tall.

The western oak may appear as a bundle or clump of plants, with many stems rising from one root system. The term "poison oak" is misleading; the plant is not an oak but its leaves may resemble those of an oak.

The leaves of these plants vary greatly, even on the same plant sometimes. The most helpful distinguishing feature is the leaflets, of which there are three. The upper surface of the leaf has a glossy, waxy appearance and is dark green. The lower surface may be lighter green with fine hairs in some cases. The color changes to red or orange in the fall. The flowers grow in clusters. They are small, about one-fourth inch across, white with a green tinge, and often do not develop fruit. The fruit is in clusters, white or ivory, with a green tinge, especially in the western poison oak. Each berry is slightly larger than a pea, and has surface segmental markings like that of a peeled orange. The fruit usually remains attached long after the leaves have fallen.

The poison sumac is a woody shrub or small tree, never a vine. It grows especially in swampy areas. There are 7 to 13 leaflets, each 3 to 4 inches long and 1 to 2 inches wide, without teeth on the margins. In the spring, the leaflet is bright orange. It becomes dark green later, the surface glossy above and pale green on the under side; the mid-rib is scarlet. It is orange-red or russet in the fall. The flowers are small, greenish yellow, and in clusters. The fruit is ivory or greenish, and is in loose clusters at the sides of the branches, never at the ends as in non-poisonous sumacs.

Symptoms

Onset is from a few hours to several days or more after exposure. The skin becomes red, a few small blisters appear, and usually there is itching. The involved area may increase greatly in size, with marked swelling and numerous large blisters. Fever may rise high and discomfort become great.

First aid

As soon after exposure as possible, wash the part with soap and water, then sponge it with rubbing alcohol. Following this cleansing, calamine lotion may be applied. If discomfort is not relieved, apply a wet compress, using Burow's solution diluted 1 part to about 25 parts of water, for 20-minute periods. The solution is cooling and usually gives relief.

Special First Aid Problems

Occasionally one may be faced with the necessity of caring for injuries when the victim may not react routinely. The mentally disturbed, the disoriented, the intoxicated, and those suffering from insulin reaction are among such cases. Obviously the first aid care for physical injuries remains unchanged. However, the first aider's attitude and approach to the situation require tact, diplomacy, and special regard for possible consequences. Certain characteristics may be recognized and the following information may prove helpful in handling such cases.

Mental disturbances

No first aid measures are recommended for this condition. Some symptoms are listed to help the first aider in recognizing the condition.

1. The victim may not talk, even to give his name.
2. He may be completely confused or seem stuporous.
3. He may show complete disregard for a serious in-

jury, yet complain loudly of some minor cut or bruise.

4. He may be agitated or combative.
5. Some elderly people may show great memory losses, seem to live in the past, or are indifferent to the events about them. Occasionally they may exhibit hysterical behavior.

Sometimes the victim cooperates readily and there is no special problem. Occasionally cooperation is lacking and the first aider may have difficulty in providing the needed assistance. It is for the latter cases the following suggestions are offered:

1. There is immediate need for the victim to be placed in responsible hands without delay: a law officer, relative, doctor, or ambulance crew.
2. Treat the victim with respect and patience, no matter how he reacts to you or the situation.
3. Be reassuring, and do not argue with him. Do not imply that you think he is mentally disturbed.
4. Generally avoid an authoritative, insistent, arbitrary approach. Be firm but patient. His cooperation is important.
5. If the victim seems about to commit a rash or harmful act, divert his attention in some way.
6. Only when his actions may further injure himself or others or when a life is at stake, might one be justified in physically restraining the victim.
7. It is important to have a reliable witness if you are to give first aid or otherwise help the victim. A law officer would be a first choice.

Intoxication

The first aider is likely to encounter injured people who are intoxicated. People under the influence of alcohol are relatively unable to protect themselves. For these reasons, the first aider should always check most carefully for associated injuries when dealing with the intoxicated.

The checkup for injuries presents difficulties because often the patient is uncooperative, the history he gives is often unreliable, and findings of pain and tenderness are misleading. When the first aider tests a body part for tenderness, the patient may show no reaction although an injury is present beneath the surface, but he may protest if an insignificant bruise is touched. Despite these difficulties, the first aider generally can determine what parts are injured if he is persistent and patient and if he checks and rechecks *all* the extremities, the back, and the head.

First aid.

1. If no injuries are present, ordinarily the person will sleep off the condition. Meanwhile, if the environment is cold, he should be covered sufficiently because body heat is lost rapidly in this condition, chilling is likely, and the patient is particularly susceptible to such infections as pneumonia.
2. If the person is unconscious and breathing ceases or virtually ceases, give artificial respiration while awaiting the physician or ambulance.
3. If a poisonous material such as wood alcohol or denatured alcohol has been taken, give first aid for poisoning if the patient can swallow.

Insulin reaction

Insulin means life for many diabetics. Diabetic children, as well as adults, learn to regulate the dosage well, but occasional mild reactions may occur. With unexpected activity and prolonged omission of eating, a more severe reaction results; rarely, there is great weakness, mental disturbance, convulsions, or unconsciousness. Some diabetics require no insulin; with others, the dosage is so small that severe reactions will not occur ordinarily despite unusual activity or meal changes. However, all users of insulin may be subject to insulin reaction.

The first aider should consider the possibility of insulin reaction whenever he encounters a confused, stuporous, unconscious, or mentally disturbed person if there is no other reason to account for the trouble.

Diabetics should wear a tag on a necklace or carry a card in an easily accessible place that identifies them and tells what to do in case of a reaction. Suspecting insulin reaction, the first aider should search for the tag or card **IN THE PRESENCE OF A WITNESS OR WITNESSES.**

First aid.

1. If conscious, the person usually can handle the situation alone or can direct others.
2. Look for identification (in the presence of others) and follow the directions given.
3. If identification cannot be found and the person can swallow, give him something sweet (candy, sugar, or a soft drink).
4. He should be seen by a doctor as quickly as possible.

Injuries to the eye

Injuries to the eye may be divided into three groups for first aid purposes: (1) injury to the eyelids and soft tissue about the eye, (2) injury to the surface of the eyeball, and (3) injury that extends through the surface of the eyeball into deeper tissue.

Group one cases

Injury to the eyelids is like any other soft tissue injury, and the first aid is similar; a sterile dressing and a snug bandage that encircles the head or is taped into place.

Bruises of the soft tissue beneath the eye often involve rupture of small blood vessels. Color changes then occur over several days, due to changes in chemicals liberated there, causing the familiar "black eye." Immediate cold applications tend to halt the bleeding and prevent some of the swelling. Later the application of warm wet towels will hasten absorption of the discoloring chemicals.

Group two cases

Most often in these cases, an irritating chemical splashes into the eye, or a foreign body lodges on the surface. Immediately irrigate the eye with clean water. Tilt the victim's head toward the injured side and then pour the fluid slowly into the eye while you hold the eyelids open with your fingers. The fluid should be poured into the inner corner of the eye and allowed to run over the eyeball and under the eyelids until at least a quart of water has been used. Sometimes a drinking fountain is at hand and can be used to wash out the chemical.

If a large amount of irritating material has been splashed into the eye, the irrigations should be prolonged beyond the use of a quart or so of fluid; then apply a loose dressing. Get the victim to a physician at once.

The harm from tiny foreign objects on the eye surface is not only their irritating effect but also the danger of their becoming embedded in the outer layer of the eyeball. Corneal ulcers may develop if the pupil is involved. Certain don'ts should be remembered.

1. Don't rub the eye. It drives the foreign object into the tissue and makes removal more difficult.
2. Don't examine the eye until you have washed your hands thoroughly.
3. Don't attempt to remove a foreign body with a match, toothpick, or other instrument.
4. Don't fail to get the victim to the physician if the object is embedded in the eyeball.

Certain measures can be taken safely and they usually succeed in removing the foreign body if it is not embedded.

1. Pull down the lower lid and see if the body lies on the surface of the lid's lining. If so, it can be lifted off gently with the corner of a clean handkerchief or a piece of moist cotton wrapped around a clean toothpick. (Never use dry cotton around the eye.)
2. Grasp the lashes of the upper lid gently between the thumb and forefinger while the victim looks upward. Pull the upper lid forward and down over the lower eyelid. A foreign body on the lining of the upper lid can be dislodged and swept away with the tears.

3. Flush the eye with a solution of boric acid (½ teaspoon to a glass of boiled water). This can be done with an eyedropper or a small bulb syringe.

Sometimes a person feels that a foreign body is in his eye, but none can be seen. There may be an injury without a foreign body present, for example, contact with a twig or the like or even infection. In these cases, get medical attention.

Group three cases

These are extremely serious. The object may penetrate a fraction of an inch into the eyeball—a splinter of wood or steel, a barley beard, BB shot, or a piece of glass. In any such case, there is danger that some loss of vision may result.

Make no attempt to remove the object. Apply a sterile compress or a clean cloth. Cover it with a loose bandage. Transport the victim *flat,* using a stretcher. The sooner the victim gets medical care, the greater the chance of saving his sight.

CHAPTER XIV

SKELETAL INJURIES

Although fractures are classified broadly as simple (closed) and compound (open), there are many variations within these two kinds. For example, if a bone is broken straight across, it is called a transverse fracture; if the break runs obliquely, it is an oblique fracture. Sometimes when force is applied to a bone, the bone bends somewhat and splits part-way down its long axis, just as a green stick does when bent. This is called a green stick fracture. It occurs most often in children, because their bones are not brittle. Green stick fractures require immobilization as a first aid measure. These fractures present only minimum evidence of soreness and tenderness to the touch.

Some muscles such as those of the heart and stomach contract without our voluntary control. Most other muscles are subject to our will, and extend from one bone to another, attaching the two bones. When they contract, they cause bending at the intervening joint. If a bone is broken, the adjacent muscles go into spasm. This action has some protective effect. The tissue in the area seems harder than usual and better able to withstand pressure or a blow.

However, the spasm also has the effect of pulling upon

the broken bone parts, causing them to overlap each other. The amount of overlap, or overriding, varies with such factors as the specific bone and the elapsed time. Bone ends in the finger may override only a fraction of an inch, whereas in the thigh, overriding is often two inches or more. Most of the overriding occurs at once because of the muscle action but in many cases, it increases slowly over several hours.

Obviously, the muscle spasm causes the broken ends to dig into the soft tissue and injure it. Muscles, blood vessels, and nerves may be affected. Motion by the victim or movement in association with transportation increases the overriding and the injury. The usual methods described in the standard section keep the parts quiet and thus prevent the sharp bone ends from stabbing motions, but they do not counteract the spasm itself.

Overriding is not a problem with fractures of certain bones, because the bones are not subject to muscle action or because of the bone construction and the manner of muscle attachments. Examples are the skull, face bones, ribs, backbone, pelvis, fingers, toes, palm, and foot bones. It is most important with the long bones of the extremities, especially the thigh and shin bone, because of strong muscle attachments. Traction splinting is a counteracting measure. The application of this type of splint is described in another section. Although it does not significantly decrease overriding already present with thigh or shin bone fractures, it lessens additional progress and relieves spasm and pain. The method is superior to ordinary splinting for fractures of these bones except when the break is within about an inch of the ankle.

It is particularly worthwhile if lengthy transportation or transportation over rough terrain is necessary. First aiders should remember that splinting is easy; it is cheap insurance.

Fracture of the Skull — Concussion of the Brain

The brain lies in a rigid compartment. If it is injured, there is only limited space for swelling. Nevertheless, the heart must pump blood into the area to sustain life.

Following a severe injury to the brain, a series of symptoms and signs appear as the tissue bleeds and swells and the heart tries to pump enough blood to the injured, compressed brain parts. Unconsciousness may occur immediately after the injury. It may last only a few seconds or many hours. Sometimes it is delayed a half-hour or more; in such cases, slow bleeding is probably present.

Symptoms. When the head sustains a blow, the brain is propelled against the skull. If the injury is minor, headache may be the only symptom. If it is extensive, unconsciousness develops. In some cases, the heart pumps blood to the injured head by powerful, slow contractions. In these cases the pulse is full and slow, the facial color reddish-purple, the breathing heavy, and the blood pressure high. In other cases of brain injury and unconsciousness, or at a later stage following the slow, full pulse, the brain is so badly injured that nerve messages to the heart and other factors governing its action are affected. The heartbeat then is weak and rapid, the face color ashen, the breathing labored, and the blood pressure low.

If the under part of the skull is broken, there may be blood, possibly only a few drops in an ear canal.

Skull fracture may also be associated with mild or profuse bleeding from the nose and throat.

Whether paralysis of one or more extremities occurs or changes in the eye pupils—unequal in size, dilated, or constricted—depends upon the parts of the brain affected.

First aid.

1. Escaping blood injures nerve tissues, sometimes irreversibly. Therefore, quiet is of extreme importance: it is the only means of lessening bleeding. The victim should lie down and be kept quiet.

2. If the face is flushed, pillows should be placed under the head and shoulders; if the face is ashen, no pillows should be used. Stimulants should not be given.

When a person sustains a severe blow to the head, he often has only a headache or perhaps a few seconds of unconsciousness. He frequently dismisses attention, walks about, and seems uninjured. However, there is always the chance that evidence of serious trouble will appear later. He should lie down and remain completely quiet until medical attention is obtained.

Fractures of the Face Bones and Nose

In these cases a noticeable bruise or wound is generally present. No first aid measures are needed against the local injury except perhaps a dressing. People sometimes dismiss injuries of the nose if bleeding soon stops and the wound is small. Fracture of nasal bones frequently results in distortion unless the broken parts are properly repositioned. Such deformity may cause difficulty in breathing. Nasal bone fractures, like all others, should have medical attention.

Fracture of the Lower Jaw

In many cases, following this fracture, the teeth of the upper and lower jaws do not meet or oppose in normal fashion. There may be mild bleeding of the gum near the point of fracture because of associated injury to the soft tissue. Usually a tender spot can be located if the fingers are run along the lower margin of the jaw.

First aid. Immobilize the lower jaw against the upper jaw by an encircling bandage that extends under the chin and over the head.

Fracture of the Collarbone

This common injury results from falls upon the outstretched hand and from direct blows. The victim typically sits or stands with the shoulder bent forward, the elbow flexed, the forearm placed across the chest and supported by the hand of the opposite side. A similar position is taken often if the arm is broken. The collarbone lies just beneath the skin. Therefore, the first aider generally can detect swelling, possibly some deformity, and local tenderness by running his fingers along the bone.

First aid. If the shoulders flex forward, the broken ends tend to override more. Throwing the shoulders back corrects the overriding slightly and diminishes discomfort. The upper extremity on the same side should be supported by a full arm-sling. A narrow bandage may be used, if comfortable, to encircle the chest and affected side. Adjust the bandages or bandage so that they tend to keep the shoulders erect.

Fracture of the Spine

The vertebrae of the spine are small in comparison with the size of the body trunk; they have a part in weight-bearing and are subject to the action of powerful back muscles. It is not surprising that spine injuries are common. Strenuous muscle action, such as lifting, may strain back muscles, cause discs to slip from normal position, and even cause fracture. Sometimes a vertebra is broken when a person lands upon his feet after a fall. Many spinal fractures result from violent forward flexion, as in falls and when an automobile occupant is thrown forward suddenly because of a collision. Neck fractures may occur when diving into shallow water.

An individual vertebra contains a central part, or body, and bone processes extending from the part. Sometimes the central part is merely compressed; this is called a compression fracture even though there is not a break line. The patient with a compression fracture must remain in a body cast with his back hyperextended for a long time so that the vertebra gradually returns to normal shape. During such first aid procedures as transportation, the preferred position likewise is with hyperextension of the back rather than forward flexion.

Looking at a vertebra from the top rather than side, one can see that there is an opening through it. The large nerve from the brain (the spinal cord) extends down the spine through these openings in the vertebrae. In case of a spine fracture or displacement, there may be pressure against the spinal cord, or sometimes the cord may be severed. In such case, there is partial or complete paralysis involving body parts whose nerve supply is cut off. Most back injuries do not cause paralysis. The danger is greatest with fractures or dislocation of neck vertebrae, though it is present when other vertebrae are injured. If the spinal cord in the neck is injured, immediate death may result because the nerve supply from the brain to vital organs is shut off. Fractures of the neck must be handled with utmost caution, keeping the victim absolutely quiet and, if possible, summoning the physician to the scene. It is easy to see that transportation of any patient who has paralysis due to any spinal fracture is hazardous; with pressure already present against the cord, any swaying motion may cause additional pressure and cutting.

Signs and symptoms. The amount of swelling and tenderness is variable, often hardly noticeable. The victim may have considerable pain while lying quiet, but sometimes he has little discomfort except when he tries to twist his back. If the spinal cord is slightly injured in the neck region, there is tingling or numbness along the shoulder and upper extremity, and perhaps weakness of the extremity. If the cord injury is severe, all upper extremities may be paralyzed. Should the cord be injured at lower levels, the upper extremities show no paralysis; but there are unusual sensations, such as tingling and numbness involving one or both of the lower extremities, and perhaps partial or complete paralysis. Whenever a person has a pain in the back, or neck, following an accident, consider the possibility of spine fracture even though local swelling and tenderness are absent. In neck cases, the person will have pain upon turning the head; in lower back injury cases, the pain often is somewhat worse if he twists the back.

First aid. In case of neck injury, keep the person flat on his back, without pillows. His head should not tilt forward or sideways. If transportation is absolutely essential, even for a few feet, use a firm frame support. The first aider should steady the victim's head, preferably using the hands because other methods are less effective. By placing the fingers at the sides of the head just below the victim's ears and exerting traction in a straight line away from the trunk, the injured part is kept quiet and discomfort lessened. If the chest or lumbar vertebrae are injured, the victim should lie on a firm frame on his back; or if the support is less rigid, as with a stretcher, he should lie on his abdomen. If the body must be turned, it should be turned as a unit so that no twisting occurs. Obviously, jackknifing the body may cause severe additional injury. Sometimes, when a chest or lumbar spine break is present, the victim insists on lying on his side. If such is the position of comfort, the first aider can only accept the victim's wishes, cautioning him against motion.

Fracture of the Pelvis

Many fractures of the pelvis heal well if the victim is merely kept in bed. Sometimes there is damage to the socket for the thigh bone, and surgery or traction on the lower extremity is necessary. Sometimes the pelvic fracture is associated with injury to the internal organs of the digestive, urinary, or genital systems.

Signs and symptoms. Victims of pelvic fractures sometimes have no pain while lying down, but do complain when they stand and walk about. The discomfort generally is in the lower abdomen or crotch or along the crease of the groin.

First aid. If there is a possibility of pelvic bone fracture, with or without internal organ injury, the victim should lie on his back and, if necessary, be transported in this position. The knees may be flexed and pillows placed beneath them for further comfort. Should the victim complain of pain in the hip region, or of pain when starting any motion of the lower extremity, such as rotating it a bit, the extremity should be splinted. The splinting does no harm if the fracture involves the pelvic bone; it may be of great value if the thigh bone is broken.

Rib Fractures

These injuries are generally caused by blows and falls. The most common locations are the lower part of the chest in front and on the sides. Occasionally, a strong blow breaks several ribs and caves in the chest somewhat, perhaps with damage to the internal organs.

Signs and symptoms. Most often with rib fractures there is little or no noticeable swelling or deformity. The victim has pain upon deep breathing. A tender spot can be located usually by running the fingers along the ribs.

First aid. No local measures are necessary if the pain is minimal. When pain is more marked, an attempt should be made to lessen breathing movements by applying one or more wide bandages around the chest. One bandage should be at the level of the injury. If the site is not at the lower part of the chest, another bandage should be circled there because breathing movements are best controlled in this way. If the bandages cause pain, they should be removed.

In cases where the ribs seem depressed because of the injury, bandages should *not* be applied around the chest, lest the broken rib ends be driven deeper into the soft tissue.

Fractures of Finger and Thumb

There are three bones in each finger and two in the thumb. When one of these bones is broken, there is the typical evidence of some swelling, little or much deformity, and tenderness to pressure. A common injury is manifested mainly by swelling at a joint, pain, and limitation of motion. It may be caused by a blow, catching a baseball or football, or bumping the extended digit. The injury is sometimes regarded as a sprain, whereas often there is a chip fracture at the end of the bone.

Fractures of Wrist and Forearm

There are eight small bones in the wrist and two in the forearm. When the wrist bones are broken or slightly dislocated, the error of regarding the injury as a sprain is common. Forearm fractures, most often near the wrist, are exceedingly common. The fingers and thumb can be moved quite freely in case of wrist and forearm fractures; such motion may cause some discomfort in the injured area.

Fracture of Arm Bone (Humerus)

Fracture of the arm bone presents no special first aid problem except that a break near the upper end may often be overlooked. The victim, of course, has some discomfort and limits his arm motion, but may doubt at first that a break is present. One helpful procedure is to examine for tenderness of the arm on the inner aspect, at the armpit level.

Fracture of the Ankle

There are two bones in the leg, the large shinbone, or tibia, on the inner side and the thinner fibula on the outer side. A fracture at the ankle may involve the outer bone an inch or so from its lower end; in this case the swelling is on the outer side of the ankle. If the small, downward-projecting process of the shinbone may be broken off, then the swelling is on the inner side of the ankle. Sometimes the shinbone is broken completely across about an inch or two above its lower end. This serious injury is a leg fracture, but might be regarded by an inexperienced person as an ankle injury.

It is impossible to tell accurately by the amount of swelling, tenderness, and pain whether the injury is a sprain or a fracture. The use of an ankle bandage, under the impression that the injury is a sprain is often done wrongly; an X-ray should be taken before heavy weight on the part is attempted.

Fracture of the Leg

If a leg fracture is present, the first aider can generally find significant evidence. The best immobilization method, aside from traction splinting, is to apply a splint to each side of the leg. These splints should be long, extending from below the heel, almost to the groin and hips, with padding about the ankle and knee. The bottom of the foot should be at right angles to the long axis of the leg as viewed from the side. The need to prevent sagging of the foot is especially important when the break is within four or five inches of the ankle.

The shinbone lies just beneath the skin surface. Improper handling may permit the broken bone end to cut through the skin. It is also possible that despite good splinting, a broken end will cut through the skin, if the leg is subject to jostling during transportation. Traction splinting is the best immobilization method for leg fracture if the break is far enough above the ankle so that the necessary traction bandages can be applied.

Fracture of the Kneecap (Patella)

This bone may be injured by direct blows or a fall. Sometimes the break results from strong muscle action alone when the knee is partly flexed. The break is usually across the bone, not up and down. By applying a splint from the heel to the buttocks along the back of the extremity, the broken kneecap parts are kept from being pulled apart by knee flexion, and soft tissue injury is kept to a minimum.

Fracture of the Thighbone (Femur)

The thighbone has a small neck-like projection at the upper end, surmounted by a ball-like structure that fits into the socket of the pelvic bone.

Fractures of the main portion of the bone give clear-cut evidence ordinarily: The victim knows that a break is likely and will not move the part to any extent. Swelling may not be clearly evident, because there is much soft tissue in the thigh and swelling may not show through as an enlargement. Tenderness can almost always be noted. Thus, if a checkup is made, the first aider should be able to find the evidence of a break.

When a break involves the neck of the femur, as it often does with elderly people following falls, the evidence is minimal. Examination frequently cannot be done. The first aider must conclude whether to splint from study of the accident and the victim's reactions and answers. The extremity is generally rotated outward so that the toes point toward the side, but this finding does not prove fracture. The victim usually is reluctant to move the extremity and probably has some discomfort at the hip. Traction splinting is useful whether the shaft of the bone or the small upper end is broken.

CHAPTER XV

FIRST AID KITS AND SUPPLIES

From your study of first aid you have learned how to improvise a number of bandages, dressings, and splints. It is, of course, more satisfactory to have sterile dressings, prepared splints, and other first aid equipment prepared and ready for use before the accident occurs.

There are two general types of first aid kits: (1) the unit type, and (2) those in which there is little uniformity in size and type of contents.

Unit-Type Kits

These kits have a complete assortment of first aid materials put up in standard packages of unit size or multiples of the unit size and arranged in cases of 16, 24, or 32 units. Each unit package contains one or more individual dressings. Each dressing is complete in itself and is sealed in a sterile wrapper. It contains just enough material to treat a single injury, thus eliminating waste. All liquids are put up in individual, sealed glass ampoules, and consequently cannot deteriorate. There are no bottles to spill or break.

Illustrations and instructions for the use of the contents are on the front of each package. The contents are clearly indicated on the top side in bold type, which makes the desired unit packages easy to locate. The unit packages fit like blocks in the case; they cannot shift or become disarranged. This kit is probably the most satisfactory if it is to be carried in a car, truck, or pack.

Standard refills are supplied by various manufacturers and can be changed easily to meet the needs of the purchaser. Unit refills are easy to obtain. The original cost may be slightly higher, but when materials are subject to much handling by many different persons, this type is generally cheaper and more satisfactory in the long run. There is no contamination or waste of unused materials. The kits can be obtained with contents selected to meet the particular needs of the purchaser.

Other Kits

Kits commonly found in drug stores are those in which uniformity in size or type are generally lacking. These kits come in a wide range of sizes, from the small pocket kit to the large cabinet type. These kits are satisfactory if the following points are observed in their selection:

1. The kit should be large enough and have the proper contents for the place where it is to be used.
2. The contents should be arranged so that the desired package can be found quickly without unpacking the entire contents.
3. Material should be wrapped so that unused portions do not become dirty through handling.

Contents of 16-Unit First Aid Kit

2 units—1" Adhesive Compress
2 units—2" Bandage Compress
1 unit—3" Bandage Compress
1 unit—4" Bandage Compress
1 unit—3" x 3" Plain Gauze Pads
1 unit—Gauze Roller Bandage
2 units—Plain Absorbent Gauze—½ sq. yd.
2 units—Plain Absorbent Gauze—24" x 72"
3 units—Triangular Bandages
1 unit—Tourniquet—Scissors—Tweezers

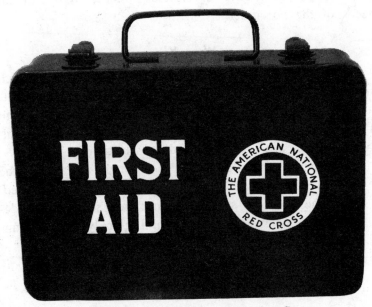

Fig. 63   16-unit first aid kit (closed).

Contents of 24-Unit First Aid Kit

2 units—1" Adhesive Compress
2 units—2" Bandage Compress
2 units—3" Bandage Compress
2 units—4" Bandage Compress
1 unit—3" x 3" Plain Gauze Pads
2 units—Gauze Roller Bandage
1 unit—Eye Dressing Packet
4 units—Plain Absorbent Gauze—½ sq. yd.
3 units—Plain Absorbent Gauze—24" x 72"
4 units—Triangular Bandages
1 unit—Tourniquet—Scissors—Tweezers

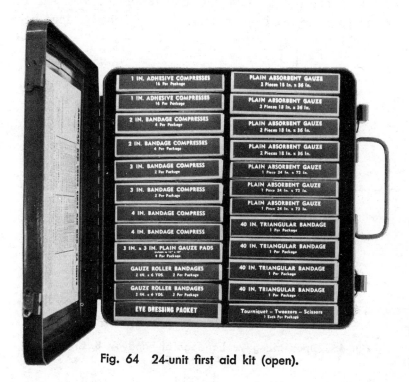

Fig. 64   24-unit first aid kit (open).

CHAPTER XVI

FIRST AID SKILLS FOR
ADVANCED COURSE

Triangular Bandage for the Hand or Foot

With the triangle spread out, place the hand with the injured side up, so that the middle of the base of the bandage comes well up on the wrist. Fold the bandage back

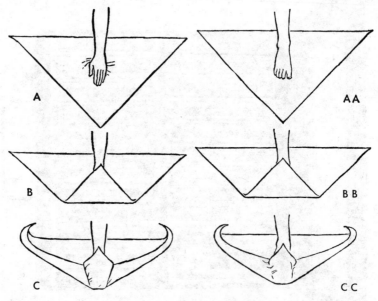

Fig. 65   Open triangular bandage of hand—A, B, C; or foot—
AA, BB, CC.

around the tips of the fingers and over the back of the hand so that the point comes well up on the wrist or forearm. Each half of the edge formed at the end of the fingers is then carried back toward the wrist, parallel to the hand, to take up slack and make a smoother bandage. Cross the ends around the wrist, tie them, and tuck them under.

Triangular Bandage for the Head

Fold a hem about 2 inches wide along the base. With the hem on the outside, place the bandage on the head so that the middle of the base lies on the forehead close down to the eyebrows and the point hangs down the back (A). Carry the two ends around the head above the ears and cross

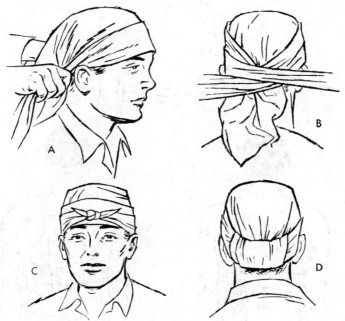

Fig. 66   Open triangular bandage for the head.

(do not tie) them just below the bump at the back of the head (B). Draw the ends snugly, carry them around the head and tie them in the center of the forehead (C). Steady the head with one hand and with the other draw the point down firmly behind to hold the compress securely against the head (D). Turn the point up and tuck it in where the bandage crosses, or pin it down with a safety pin at the back of the head.

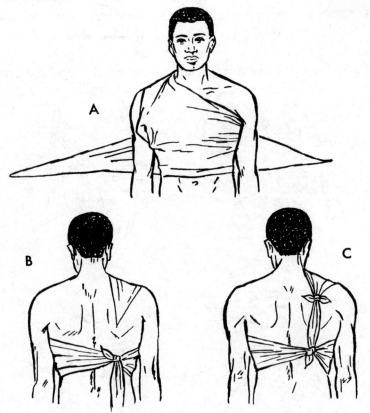

Fig. 67 Open triangular bandage for the chest or back.

Triangular Bandage for the Chest or Back

Place the point of the bandage over the shoulder on the injured side. Carry the bandage down over the chest (or back) so that the middle of the base is directly below the shoulder (A). Roll or fold the base as far up as you desire. Carry the ends around the body and tie them directly below the shoulder (B). This leaves one long and one short end. Carry the long end up to the shoulder and tie it (C).

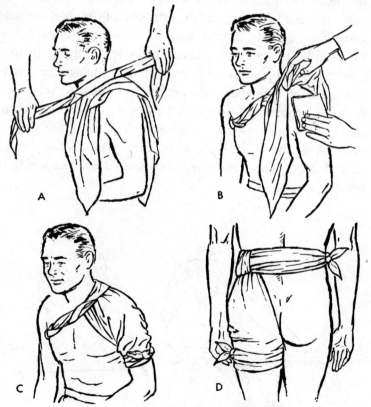

Fig. 68   Bandage for the shoulder or hip.

Triangular Bandage for Shoulder or Hip

Two triangular bandages, or one triangular bandage and a necktie or strip of cloth, are required. If two triangular bandages are used, fold one into a narrow cravat. Pin or roll the point of the second or unfolded triangular bandage around this cravat several turns to secure it (A). Pleat the unfolded triangular bandage, laying it with the middle of the folded cravat over the injured shoulder (B). Carry the end of the cravat or strip of cloth around the body below the opposite armpit and tie it slightly forward from the armpit. Unfold the pleated triangle, bringing it down over the dressing so that the base of the bandage lies on the arm. Fold the bandage up the arm as far as desired (C). Cross the ends around the arm and tie them snugly but not too tight. Check the amount of pressure by feeling the pulse at the wrist on the injured side to make sure circulation has not been shut off. The same procedure is used for bandaging the hip (D).

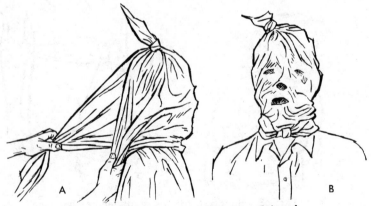

Fig. 69 Bandage for the face and head.

Triangular Bandage for the Face and/or Back of the Head

Tie a knot at the point of the bandage, beginning the knot about 6 inches from the point. Place the knot at the crown of the head. Carry the base down over the face and chin to the neck. Carry one end around to the back, covering the cheek, ear, and back of the head and neck. Carry the other end around in a like manner, crossing it over the first end. Bring the ends to the front and tie them under the chin. Cut a slit for the nose and eyes if they are not injured. The same bandage may be used to cover injuries to the back of the head, the face being left exposed.

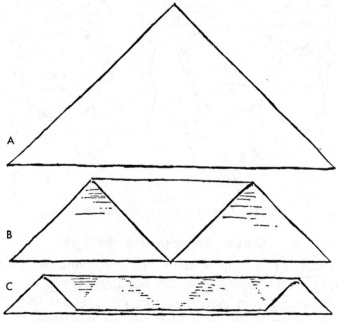

Fig. 70   Folding the triangle to make a cravat.

Triangular Bandage Folded As a Cravat

To make a cravat bring the point of a triangular bandage to the middle of the base. Then fold lengthwise along the middle until you obtain the desired width.

Cravat Bandage for Head or Ear

Place the center of the cravat over the compress covering the wound. Carry the ends around to the opposite side of the head, cross them, bring them back to the starting point and tie them.

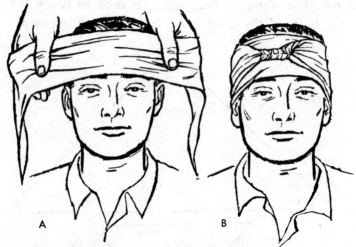

A   B

Fig. 71   Cravat bandage for the forehead.

Cravat Bandage for the Eye

Lay a thin strip of cloth over the uninjured eye (A). Place a cravat bandage over this and across the forehead over the injured eye and under the ear on the same side (B). Tie in center of the forehead (C). Using the thin strip of cloth, pull the cravat up from the uninjured eye and tie (D).

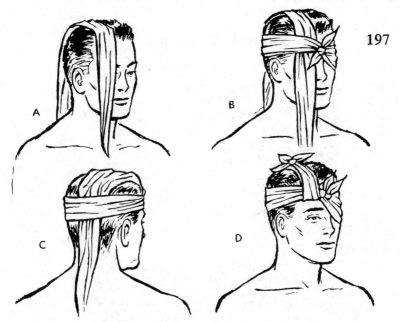

Fig. 72 Cravat bandage for the eye.

Cravat Bandage for the Neck

Place the center of the cravat over the compress covering the wound. Carry the ends around the neck, cross them at the opposite side, bring them back to the starting point, and tie them loosely.

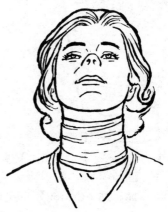

Fig. 73 Cravat bandage for the neck.

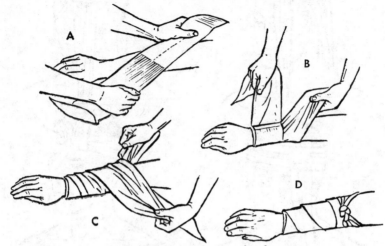

Fig. 74   Cravat bandage for the forearm.

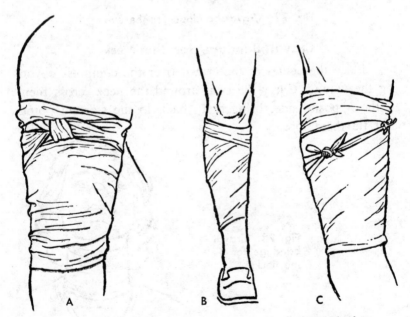

Fig. 75   Cravat bandage for A. Arm, B. Leg, C. Thigh.

Cravat Bandage for the Forearm, Arm, Leg, or Thigh

Place the end of the cravat diagonally across the part to be covered, some distance from the injury (A), and spiral the longer end around the part (B). Space the turns of the spiral so that the approximate middle of the cravat makes the turn that lies at the lower end of the part (C), then spiral it back up the part and tie the ends (D).

Cravat Bandage for Cheek or Ear

Use a wide cravat. Start with the middle of the cravat over the compress covering the cheek or ear. Carry one end over the top of the head and the other under the chin (A). Cross the ends at the opposite side (B). Bring the short end back around the forehead and the long end around the back of the head. Tie them over the compress (C).

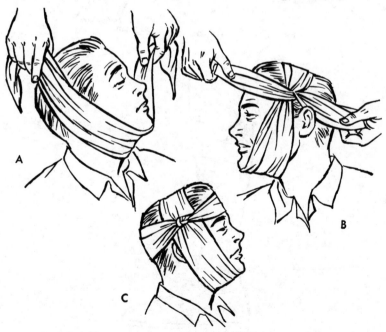

Fig. 76 Cravat bandage for cheek or ear.

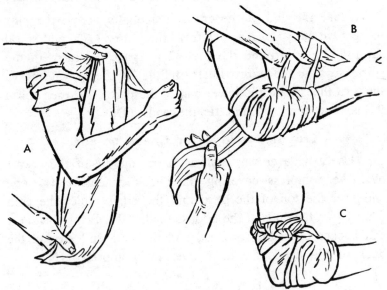

Fig. 77   Cravat bandage for elbow.

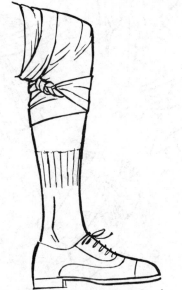

Fig. 78   Cravat bandage for knee.

Cravat Bandage for Elbow or Knee

Bend the elbow or knee at a right angle unless this movement produces pain. Use a cravat (8 inches wide or more) and place the middle over the elbow or knee. Carry the ends around, crossing them in the hollow. (A). Carry the upper end entirely around the arm or thigh above the elbow or knee and bring it back to the hollow (B). Carry the lower end entirely around the forearm or leg below the elbow or knee and bring it back to the hollow (C). Tie snugly at the outside edge of the hollow.

Cravat Bandage for the Palm of the Hand
(Figure-of-Eight)

Use a rather narrow cravat. Lay the middle of the cravat straight across the palm (A), leaving the thumb out. While holding the bandage in place, carry the end hanging

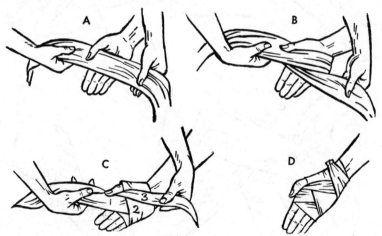

Fig. 79 Cravat bandage for palm of hand.

from the thumb side (B), diagonally around the back of the
hand, then from the heel on the little finger side diagonally
across the palm to the space between the thumb and index
finger. Take the other end and carry it around the back of
the hand to the base of the thumb (C-1), then across the
palm to the little finger side, around and across the back of
the hand (C-2), and bring it up in the crotch of the thumb,
snugging it underneath the other end at this point, and carry
it across the palm diagonally to the wrist (C-3). Finish by
carrying the other end across the back of the hand to the heel
of the little finger side, thus locking the previous turns, and
wrap both ends around the wrist and tie them (D).

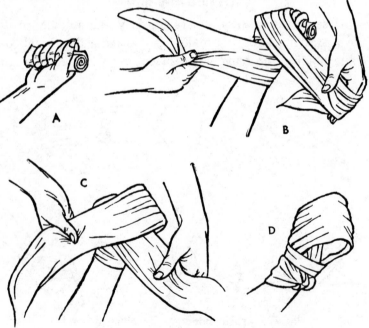

Fig. 80   Pressure bandage for palm of hand.

Pressure Bandage for the Palm

Place a sterile pad in the palm of the hand and close the fingers over it firmly (A). Lay the center of a cravat bandage over the upturned wrist. Take the end on the thumb side and bring it up over the back of the hand, opposite the thumb side and over the two fingers on that side (B). Take the other end and bring it diagonally across the back of the hand and over the other two fingers (C). The ends should cross over the upturned wrist. At this point, pull down firmly on the crossed ends to hold the fingers tightly against the pad in the palm. Cross the ends in opposite directions around the wrist and tie at the side of the wrist (D).

Temporary Bandage To Support a Sprained Ankle

Leave the shoe on. If the shoe is high-topped, loosen the laces to allow for swelling. Place the middle of a narrow cravat under the shoe just in front of the heel. Carry the ends up and back, crossing them at the back of the heel (A); continue around the ankle crossing the ends over the instep, then downward toward the arch to make a hitch under the

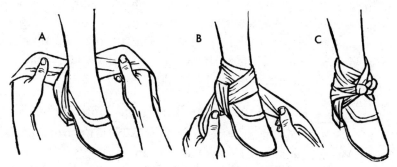

Fig. 81 Temporary support for sprained ankle.

cravat on each side, in front of the heel. Pull the ends in opposite directions (B) to achieve the desired tension. Cross the ends over the instep and tie them (C).

Spiral Reverse Bandage of the Limbs

Because the limbs are tapered, a spiral bandage must include an occasional reverse-lap to overcome gaps or open spaces in the bandage. Anchor the bandage with two or three turns around the small part of the limb (A). Then start wrapping with a spiral turn as long as each turn will lie

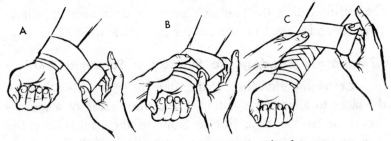

Fig. 82   Spiral reverse bandage for the forearm.

flat and overlap the preceding turn by at least one-third the width of the bandage (B). When a gap develops, it requires use of a "reverse." This is done by holding the lower edge of the last turn that fits properly, then loosely making a neat half-twist (C) or lap to change slightly the direction of the spiral. Continue the spiral wraps up the limb, repeating the "reverse" each time it is needed.

Figure-of-Eight Bandage for Hand and Wrist

Anchor the bandage with one or two turns around the palm of the hand, then carry it diagonally across the front of the wrist, and around the wrist (A). Again carry it di-

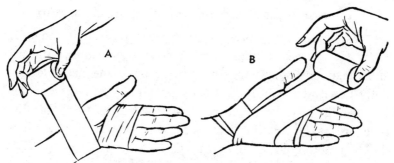

Fig. 83   Figure-of-eight bandage for the hand and wrist.

agonally across the front of the wrist (B), and back to the palm. This figure-of-eight maneuver is repeated as many times as is necessary to fix the dressing properly.

Figure-of-Eight Bandage for the Ankle

Start the bandage on the instep and take two or three anchoring turns around the instep and foot (A). Carry the bandage diagonally upward across the front of the foot, then around the ankle (B) and diagonally downward across the front of the foot and across under the arch. Several of these figure-of-eight turns are made, each turn overlapping the previous one by about two-thirds the width of the bandage (C). Occasionally use an extra turn around the ankle.

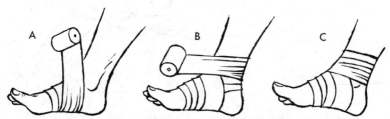

Fig. 84   Figure-of-eight bandage for the ankle.

Figure-of-Eight Bandage for Neck and Armpit

Make two or more anchoring wraps around the arm (A). Carry the bandage from under the armpit, upward and diagonally across the shoulder, around the neck, diagonally downward, across the same shoulder, and then under the armpit (B). A number of figure-of-eight turns of this type are taken so that by overlapping you can cover the dressing and hold it in place (C).

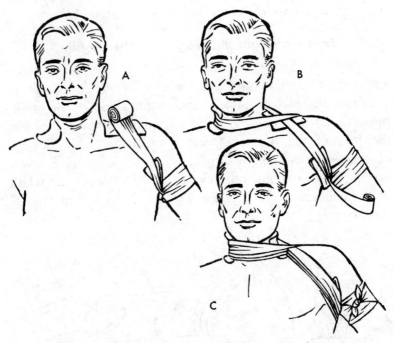

Fig. 85   Figure-of-eight bandage for neck and armpit.

Four-Tail Bandage

The appearance of this bandage gives it its name. Because a pocket can be formed by crossing the tails in pairs when tying the bandage, it fits particularly well over protuberances such as the nose and chin. A piece of cloth about 3 feet long and from 3 to 8 inches wide is split from each end down the middle, leaving as large a center area as is needed. Gauze may be used, but heavier cloth is more satisfactory. First apply a dressing over the wound, then center the bandage over it (A and C). Carry the upper pair of tails downward and the lower pair of tails upward to tie

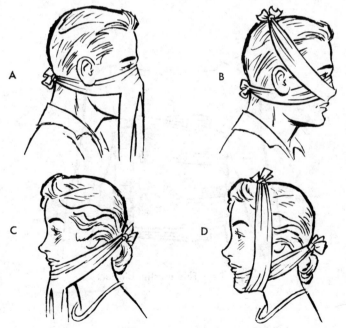

Fig. 86   Four-tail bandage of nose (A, B) and chin (C, D).

the bandage so that it fits smoothly (B and D). This bandage may be used for wounds of the nose, chin, and lower jaw. IT SHOULD NOT BE USED FOR A FRACTURE OF THE JAW.

Muslin Binder

When bulky dressings are needed for wounds of the abdomen or chest, the simplest form of bandage is usually a binder, made from a rectangular piece of cloth about 12 to 18 inches wide and 3 to 5 feet long. The binder is placed around the back and pinned in front. A large bath towel makes a good binder.

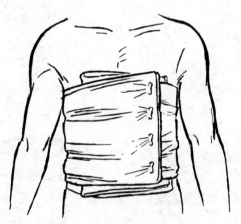

Fig. 87 The muslin binder.

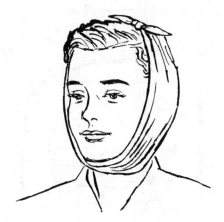

Fig. 88   Bandage for Fracture of Lower Jaw.

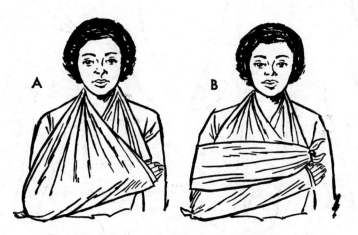

Fig. 89   Bandages for Fracture of Collarbone.

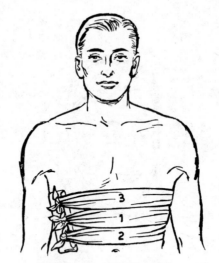

Fig. 90   Rib Fracture.

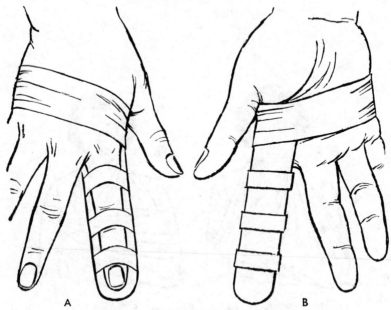

A   B

Fig. 91   Splint for Broken Finger.

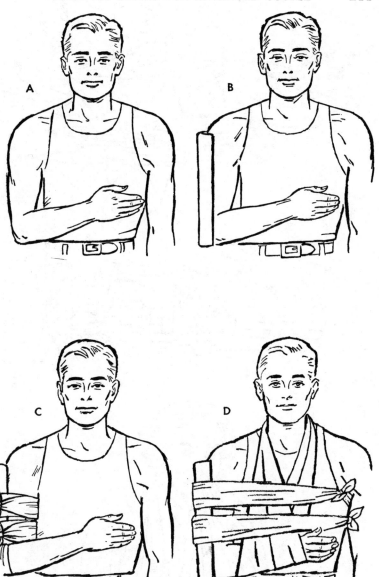

Fig. 92   Splint for Fracture of Armbone.

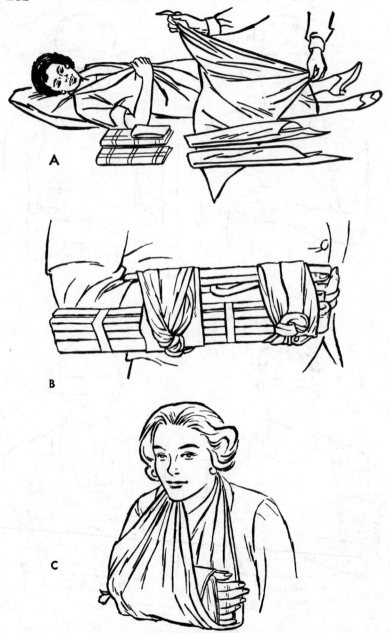

Fig. 93 Splint for Forearm and Wrist.

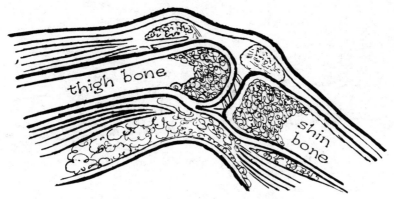

Fig. 94   Fractured Knee Cap.

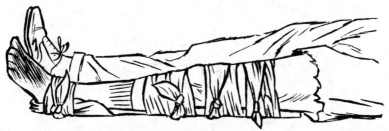

Fig. 95   Fixation Splint of Knee Cap.

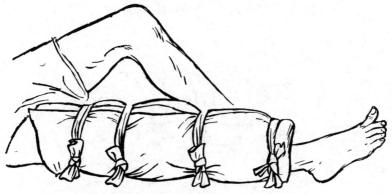

Fig. 96   Improvised Splint of Knee Cap.

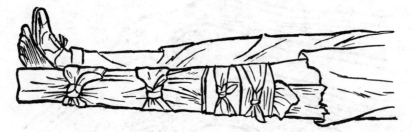

Fig. 97—Fixation Splint—Fracture of Leg.

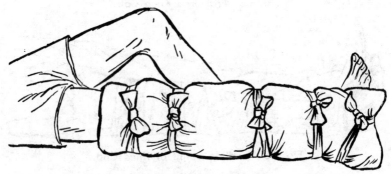

Fig. 98   Improvised Splint—Fracture of Leg.

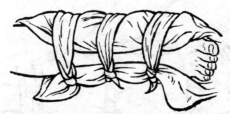

Fig. 99   Splint for Crushed Foot or Toes.

Lock Hitch for Half-Ring Traction Splint

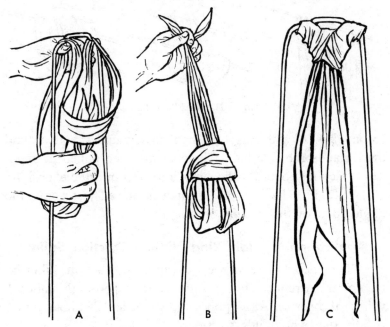

Fig. 100   Lock Hitch for Half-Ring Traction Splint.

Make a cravat bandage. Bring the two ends together and lay the loop over the end of the splint (A). Bring the two tails through the loop (B) and pull downward to tighten (C). Make sure the ends of the bandage are of equal length.

Cradle Hitch

Hang the cravat over the outside bar, with the center of the cravat over the bar (A). Pass the end nearest the leg under the leg, up between the leg and the inside bar (B). The

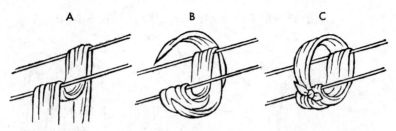

Fig. 101   Cradle Hitch.

second half of the cravat is then passed under and around the leg and both side bars. The ends are then pulled in opposite directions to bring the limb into a comfortable position (C). NOTE: The first cradle hitch is placed just above the ankle to take the weight off the limb.

Application of Half Ring Hinged Traction Splint

Two people are needed to apply a traction splint to the lower extremity. For identification purposes Number 1 will be the person who applies the splint and Number 2 will be the one who holds traction.

1. Number 2 grasps the foot of the limb to be splinted with one hand over the instep and the other hand at the heel (see drawing Fig. 102A), and exerts a strong, steady pull. He maintains this strong, steady pull until the limb is splinted. This is manual traction.

2. Number 1 fashions a lock hitch on the end of the splint (Fig. 100).

3. Flatten the half ring on the splint and place it underneath the injured limb with the "long" side at the outer side of the limb and the half ring at the buttocks.

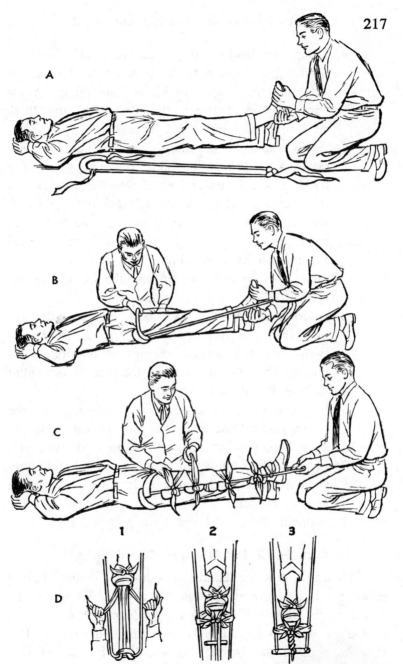

Fig. 102   Application of Half-Ring Hinged Traction Splint.

4. Using the buckle straps, lift the half ring into place against the buttocks and secure the buckle. (Note: The strap should not be tight. Allow enough room between the strap and the thigh to easily pass your hand through.)

5. Apply the ankle bandage (sprained ankle bandage). This should be snug but not tight. The bandage should be as free of wrinkles as possible.

6. Pass the ends of the lock hitch *downward* through the stirrups of the ankle bandage, and pull both ends toward Number 2 until you have equalled the tension he is holding.

7. Quickly whip the ends around the outside of the splint and tie over the center.

8. Insert a short, stout stick between the ends running from the end of the splint to the foot, and twist until the desired amount of traction is attained. Then tie the stick to the side of the splint so that it will not unwind.

9. If gauze roller bandages are available, wrap the entire limb. Otherwise use four cravat bandages as a hammock to support the injured extremity.

10. Place a block under the end of the splint to prevent the heel from coming in contact with the ground or cot.

11. Number 2 now releases manual traction.

Lock Hitch for Notched Board Splint

To attach traction bands to a notched board, fold a cravat bandage in the middle and lay about 8 inches of this fold through the notch (A). Open the loop at the fold and double the open loop back over the ends of the notch (B). Pull the ends of the cravat until the loop is snug (C).

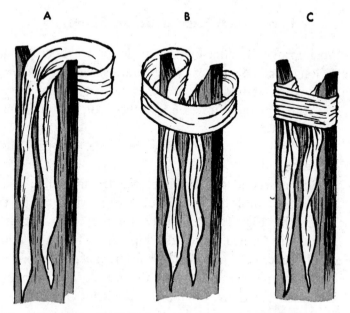

Fig. 103   The lock-hitch for notched board splint.

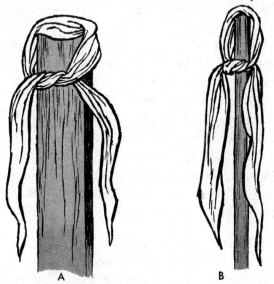

Fig. 104   A. The lock-hitch for plain board.
B. For rounded stick.

Improvised Fixed Traction Splint

An improvised splint can be made with a board about 5 feet long and 4 inches wide and ½ inch thick. A V-shaped notch should be cut in each end of the board.

1. Apply manual traction on the foot, as previously described.
2. Put on a sprained ankle bandage, as previously described.
3. Slip a second cravat under the leg and slide it up the leg until the center of the bandage is in the crotch (Fig. 103-A). Then tie the ends so that a loop is formed above the hip into which the notch of the upper end of the board is placed. Secure the cravat in the notch with the tails of the bandage.
4. Insert the tails of the lock hitch (Fig. 103-B) downward through the stirrups of the sprained ankle bandage and pass them over and under the board, and tie.
5. Insert a stout, strong stick between the traction bands below the foot and twist until you have taken up any slack left while tying the traction bands around the splint (Fig. 103-C).
6. Padding should be placed between the leg and the board wherever pressure occurs.
7. Several *wide* cravats should be wrapped around the limb and board from the ankle to the upper thigh.
8. Support the end of the splint so that the heel does not come in contact with the ground.

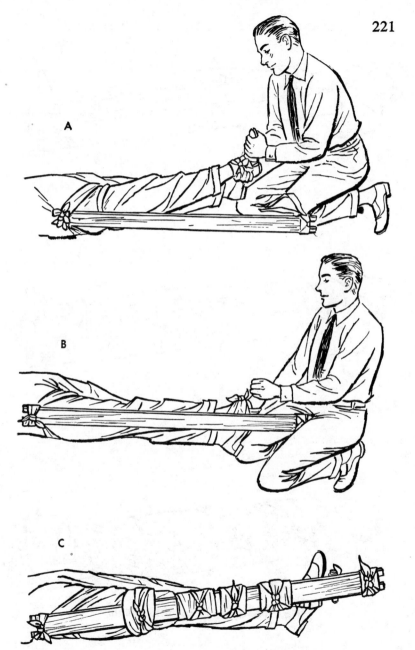

Fig. 105   Improvised Fixed Traction Splint.

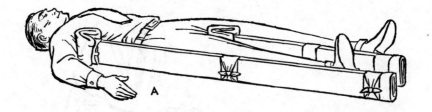

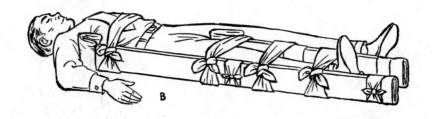

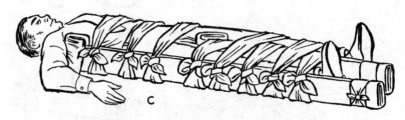

Fig. 106   Fixation Splint for Thigh.

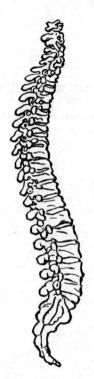

Fig. 107 The spinal column—side view.

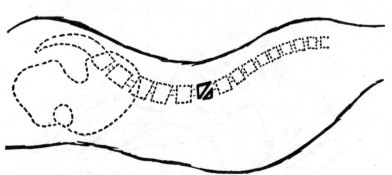

Fig. 108 Spinal Fracture.

Transportation of Victim with Suspected Neck Fracture

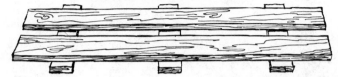

Fig. 109   Two boards used to immobilize a broken neck.

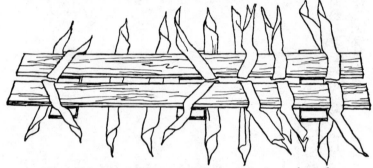

Fig. 110   Attachments for securing victim to boards.

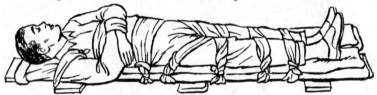

Fig. 111   Victim secured to boards.

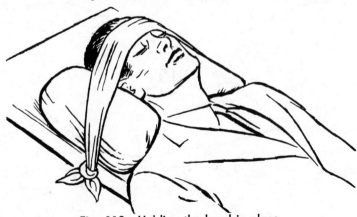

Fig. 112   Holding the head in place.

Litters and Carries

The litter shown in Fig. 113 is generally known as the army litter and is most satisfactory for general use. The litter can be loaded in many ways described in the standard section of this text.

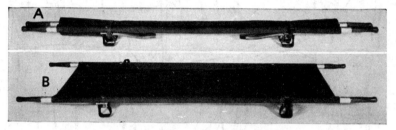

Fig. 113   Standard Army Litter.

Carrying with a litter

It is best to have four bearers: one at the head and one at the foot facing each other, and one on each side facing each other. All assume the proper lifting stance (Fig. 114) and at the command "LIFT," all stand erect. If the victim is to be carried feet first, the two bearers at the side move down to the foot of the litter and hold the load while the bearer at the foot reverses his position. If the victim is to be carried head first, the opposite action takes place. The two bearers at the side return to their normal position, make a half-turn to face the proper direction. They hold the sides of the litter with the nearest (inside) hand and

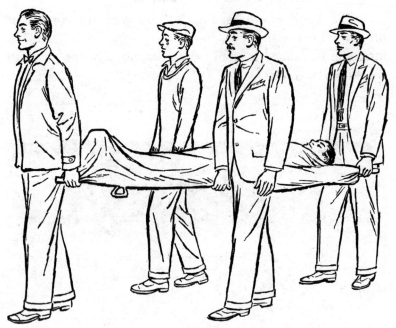

Fig. 114 Carrying a litter.

are prepared to walk forward. At the command "MARCH," the bearer at the head steps off on his *right* foot, and the bearers at the sides and foot step off on the *left* foot. To lower the litter, the steps used to lift the litter are merely reversed.

Improvised litters

When two poles are available, you can use a blanket, robe, rug, or strong double sheet as shown in Fig. 115. Make sure the material is wide enough.

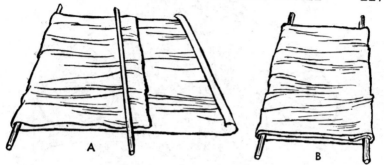

Fig. 115   Improvised litter.

Eight-man carry on the hands

Four bearers on each side kneel on the knee nearest the victim's feet. Hands, wrists, and forearms are worked gently under the victim's back until the palms of the hands are about at the midline of the back (Fig. 116). The hands should be alternated from the two sides. The two hands under the victim's head may have the fingers interlocked to form a cup for the head.

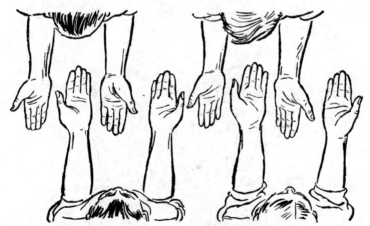

Fig. 116   Position of hands for eight-man lift and carry.

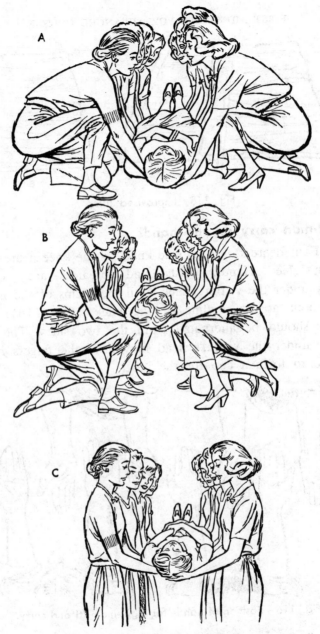

Fig. 117 The eight-man lift and carry.

At the command "LIFT," the victim is lifted on the hands and forearms to the bearers' knees (Fig. 117-B). Be careful to keep the victim's body in a straight line. At the command "STAND," the bearers stand erect (Fig. 117-C).

To lower the victim to the ground reverse the procedure.

Suspension lift—victim prone

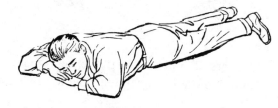

Fig. 118.1

Step 1. The victim lies in a prone position with the hands under the chin, similar to the position assumed in artificial respiration.

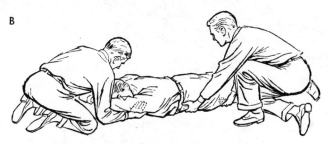

Fig. 118.2

Step 2. Carrier 1 kneels on one or both knees at the victim's head. He carefully slides his hands under the mid-forearms of the victim until the upturned palms of the hands rest under the victim's armpits.

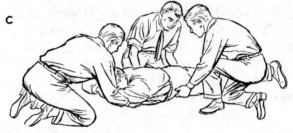

Fig. 118.3

Step 3. Carriers 2 and 3 grasp the hipbone with the top hand and the knee cap with the lower hand.

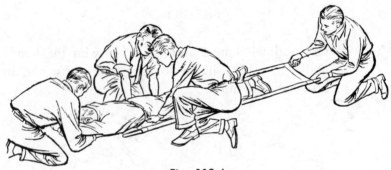

Fig. 118.4

Step 4. On signal, all lift together so that the victim is raised five or six inches from the floor (just high enough to slide a litter underneath).

NOTE: Care should be taken so that the body is lifted as a unit.

Chair carry

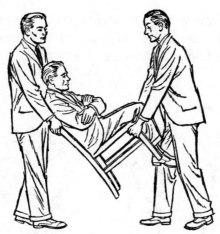

Fig. 119

A convenient technique for carrying a person when a litter is not available is to seat the victim on a strong chair, as shown above. This is also good for going up and down stairs, through narrow corridors, etc.

Carry by extremities

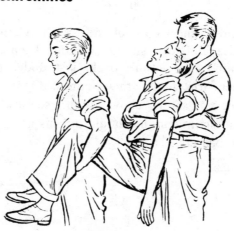

Fig. 120

This technique shown in Fig. 120 is also called the "fore and aft" carry. Its chief use is in cases of fainting or similar conditions and where there are no serious injuries to the body.

Two-man carry

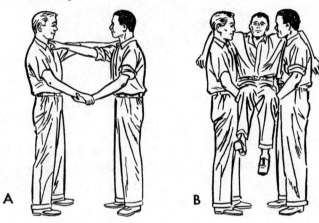

A   B

Fig. 121

The bearers kneel on each side of the victim, near his hips, and raise him to a sitting position. Then each passes one arm around the victim's back, just under the armpit, and the other arm under the victim's thighs. Grasp the wrists and neck as shown above. Both rise slowly from the ground. If the victim can, he should put his arms around the necks of the bearers.

Pack-strap carry

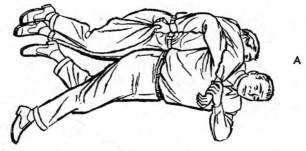

Fig. 122.A

This carry is valuable if the victim's injuries will permit its use and the victim's weight is equal to or less than that of the bearer. If the victim is lying down and cannot help, the bearer must also lie down with his back against the victim's chest. In this position reach over the victim and bring his top arm over your shoulder and hold it in place with your hand close to your chest. Grasp the clothing of the victim at his hip with the other hand and roll him over on top of you (Fig. 122-A). From this position get to both knees (Fig. 122-B), then to one knee, then stand upright (Fig. 122-C). If need be, the transfer from a walking assist to the pack-strap carry is made easily.

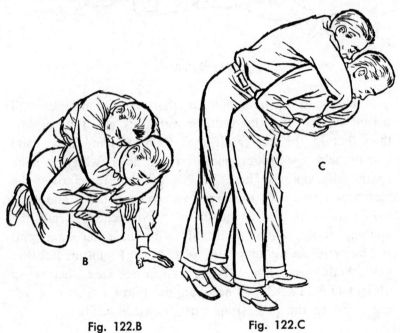

Fig. 122.B   Fig. 122.C

INDEX

Accidents, 4, 5
  cost, 5
  prevention, 5
  rate, 4
Anatomy, 134-143
Animal bites, 147-151
  danger of rabies, 147, 148
  first aid, 147
  snake, 148-151
Ankle, sprained, 203, 204
Antidotes for poisons, 51-54
  carbolic acid, 53
  if victim is in coma, 54
  kerosene, 54
  lye, 53, 54
  strychnine, 53, 54
  universal, 53
    exceptions to, 53, 54
Apoplexy (stroke), 88, 89
  first aid, 89
  symptoms, 88, 89
Appendicitis, 158
  first aid, 158
  symptoms, 158
Arm sling, 112
Arteries, 137
Artificial respiration, 32-46, 117-125
  adults, 117-121
    technique for using back-pressure-arm lift method, 117-121
  breathing process explained, 32, 33
  definition, 32
  infants and small children, techniques, 122-124

mouth-to-mouth, 125
objective in treatment, 32
resuscitators, use of, 45, 46
when arms are fractured, 125
when chest cage is impaired, 125
when to use,
  chest compression, 34
  choking and strangling, 34
drowning, 34, 45
drug poisoning, 34
electric shock, 34-38
gas poisoning, 34, 40
intoxication, 168
Backbone, anatomy, 135, 136, 223
Bandage, 103-112, 190-218
  adhesive compress, 109
  anchoring, 103
  ankle, 203-205
  armpit, 206
  arm-sling, 112
  bandage compress, 109, 110
  circular turn, 105
  collarbone, fracture, 209
  cradle hitch, 215, 216
  cravat, 196-202
  figure-of-eight, 201, 202, 205, 206
  figure-of-eight turns, 106, 107
  four-tail, 207, 208
  gauze roller, 110, 111
  gauze squares, 108, 109
  hand, 204, 205
  lock-hitch, 215, 218
  lower jaw, fracture, 209

[235]

APPENDIX A

ARTIFICIAL RESPIRATION

This appendix supersedes material on pages 117-125.

The National Academy of Sciences-National Research Council Ad Hoc Committee on Artificial Respiration in its meeting of 3 November 1958 reviewed the data on artificial respiration obtained through research projects supported by the Department of the Army, the American National Red Cross, and others.

It was unanimously agreed by members of the Ad Hoc group that the mouth-to-mouth (or mouth-to-nose) technique of artificial respiration is the most practical method for emergency ventilation of an individual of any age who has stopped breathing, in the absence of equipment or of help from a second person, regardless of the cause of cessation of breathing.

First aid-trained people do not usually have the experience, training, and essential equipment to distinguish whether or not lack of breathing is a result of disease or accident. **Therefore, some form of artificial respiration should be started at the earliest possible moment.**

Any procedure that will obtain and maintain an open air passageway from the lungs to the mouth and provide for an alternate increase and decrease in the size of the chest, internally or externally, will move air in and out of a nonbreathing person.

The mouth-to-mouth (or mouth-to-nose) technique has the advantage of providing pressure to inflate the victim's lungs immediately. It also enables the rescuer to obtain more accurate information on the volume, pressure, and timing of efforts needed to inflate the victim's lungs than are afforded by other methods.

When a person is unconscious and not breathing, the base of the tongue tends to press against and block the upper air passageway. The procedures described below should provide for an open air passageway when a lone rescuer must perform artificial respiration.

242

Mouth-to-Mouth (Mouth-to-Nose) Method
of Artificial Respiration

If there is foreign matter visible in the mouth, wipe it out quickly with your fingers or a cloth wrapped around your fingers.

1. Tilt the head back so the chin is pointing upward (Fig. 1). Pull or push the jaw into a jutting-out position (Fig. 2 and Fig. 3).

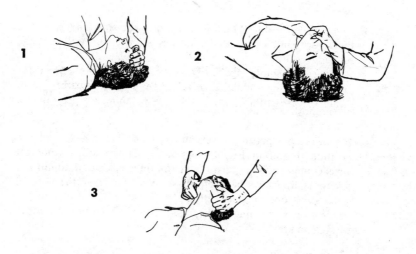

These maneuvers should relieve obstruction of the airway by moving the base of the tongue away from the back of the throat.

2. Open your mouth wide and place it tightly over the victim's mouth. At the same time pinch the victim's nostrils shut (Fig. 4) or close the nostrils with your cheek (Fig. 5). Or close the victim's mouth and place your mouth over the nose (Fig. 6). Blow into the victim's mouth or nose. (Air may be blown through the victim's teeth, even though they may be clenched.)
The first blowing efforts should determine whether or not obstruction exists.

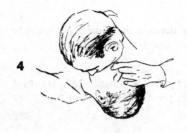

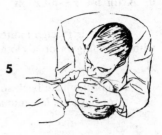

3. Remove your mouth, turn your head to the side, and listen for the return rush of air that indicates air exchange. Repeat the blowing effort.

For an adult, blow vigorously at the rate of about 12 breaths per minute. For a child, take relatively shallow breaths appropriate for the child's size, at the rate of about 20 per minute.

4. If you are not getting air exchange, recheck the head and jaw position (Fig. 1 or Fig. 2 and Fig. 3). If you still do not get air exchange, quickly turn the victim on his side and administer several sharp blows between the shoulder blades in the hope of dislodging foreign matter (Fig. 7).

Again sweep your fingers through the victim's mouth to remove foreign matter.

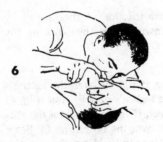

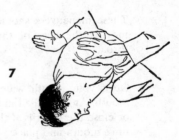

Those who do not wish to come in contact with the person may hold a cloth over the victim's mouth or nose and breathe through it. The cloth does not greatly affect the exchange of air.

Mouth-to-Mouth Technique for Infants
and Small Children

If foreign matter is visible in the mouth, clean it out quickly as described previously.

1. Place the child on his back and use the fingers of both hands to lift the lower jaw from beneath and behind, so that it juts out (Fig. 8).
2. Place your mouth over the child's mouth AND nose, making a relatively leakproof seal, and breathe into the child, using shallow puffs of air (Fig. 9). The breathing rate should be about 20 per minute.

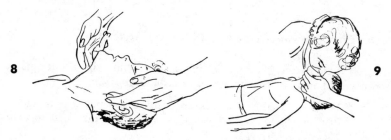

If you meet resistance in your blowing efforts, recheck the position of the jaw. If the air passages are still blocked, the child should be suspended momentarily by the ankles (Fig. 10) or inverted over one arm (Fig. 11) and given two or three sharp pats between the shoulder blades, in the hope of dislodging obstructing matter.

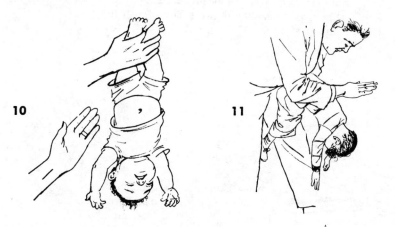

Manual Methods of Artificial Respiration

Rescuers who cannot, or will not, use mouth-to-mouth or mouth-to-nose techniques, should use a manual method. The rescuer should not be limited to the use of a single manual method for all cases, since the nature of the injury in any given case may prevent the use of one method, while favoring another.

It has already been pointed out that the base of the tongue tends to press against and block the air passage when a person is unconscious and not breathing. **This action of the tongue can occur whether the victim is in a face-down or face-up position.**

The Chest Pressure-Arm Lift (Silvester) Method

If there is foreign matter visible in the mouth, wipe it out quickly with your fingers or a cloth wrapped around your fingers.

1. Place the victim in a face-up position and put something under his shoulders to raise them and allow the head to drop backward (Fig. 12).

2. Kneel at the victim's head, grasp his arms at the wrists, cross them, and press them over the lower chest (Fig. 13). This should cause air to flow out.

3. Immediately release this pressure and pull the arms outward and upward over his head and backward as far as possible (Fig. 14). This should cause air to rush in.

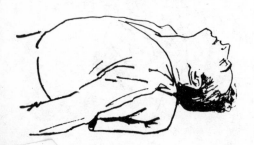
12

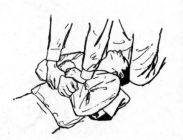
1

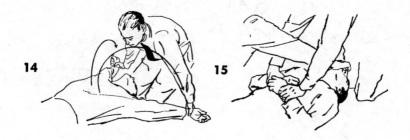

14

15

4. Repeat this cycle about 12 times per minute, checking the mouth frequently for obstructions.

   When the victim is in a face-up position, there is always danger of aspiration of vomitus, blood, or blood clots. This hazard can be reduced by keeping the head extended and turned to one side. If possible, the head should be a little lower than the trunk. If a second rescuer is available, have him hold the victim's head so that the jaw is jutting out (Fig. 15). The helper should be alert to detect the presence of any stomach contents in the mouth and keep the mouth as clean as possible at all times.

The Back Pressure-Arm Lift (Holger-Nielsen) Method

If there is foreign matter visible in the mouth, wipe it out quickly with your fingers or a cloth wrapped around your fingers.

1. Place the victim face-down, bend his elbows and place his hands one upon the other, turn his head slightly to one side and extend it as far as possible, making sure that the chin is jutting out (Fig. 16).

2. Kneel at the head of the victim. Place your hands on the flat of the victim's back so that the palms lie just below an imaginary line running between the armpits (Fig. 17).

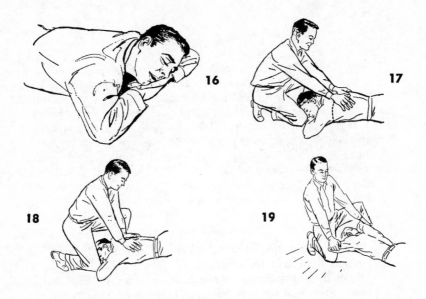

3. Rock forward until the arms are approximately vertical and allow the weight of the upper part of your body to exert steady, even pressure downward upon the hands (Fig. 18).

4. Immediately draw his arms upward and toward you, applying enough lift to feel resistance and tension at his shoulders (Fig. 19). Then lower the arms to the ground. Repeat this cycle about 12 times per minute, checking the mouth frequently for obstruction.

If a second rescuer is available, have him hold the victim's head so that the jaw continues to jut out (Fig. 20). The helper should be alert to detect any stomach contents in the mouth and keep the mouth as clean as possible at all times.

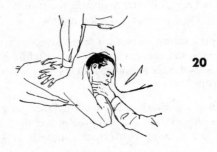

Artificial Respiration for Water Cases

Individuals who die as a result of a water accident usually die from the lack of air, and not because of water in the lungs or stomach.

A drowning victim may be either active or passive. Unless unconscious, the drowning victim usually struggles to remain on the surface or to regain the surface, in order to secure air. These efforts are energy-consuming and may result in the victim swallowing varying quantities of water. This water, along with food remaining in the stomach, could, if regurgitated, obstruct the air passages and interfere with the efforts of the rescuer. The possibility of obstruction must be recognized by the rescuer and immediate steps taken to relieve it if it occurs.

Evaporation of water from the victim's skin will result in lowering still further a body temperature that may already be dangerously low. It is imperative, therefore, to keep the victim from becoming chilled.

Related Information for All Methods

Time your efforts to coincide with victim's first attempt to breathe for himself.

If vomiting occurs, quickly turn the victim on his side, wipe out the mouth, and then reposition him.

Normally, recovery should be rapid, except in electric shock, drug poisoning, or carbon monoxide poisoning cases. In these instances, nerves and muscles controlling the breathing system are paralyzed or deeply depressed, or the carbon monoxide has displaced oxygen in the blood stream over a period of time. When these cases are encountered, artificial respiration must often be carried on for long periods.

When a victim is revived, he should be kept as quiet as possible until he is breathing regularly. He should be kept covered and otherwise treated for shock until suitable transportation is available, if he must be moved.

Artificial respiration should be continued until the victim begins to breathe for himself, or until a physician pronounces the victim dead, or until the person appears to be dead beyond any doubt.

A doctor's care is necessary during the recovery period, as respiratory and other disturbances may develop as an aftermath.

95-100 A
89-94 B+
84-88 B
80-83 B-
76-79 C+
70-75 C
64-69 C-
58-63 D+
54-57 D
50-53 D-

50 below F

437
593 pass

346 to pass